Qigong

and the

Tai Chi

Axis

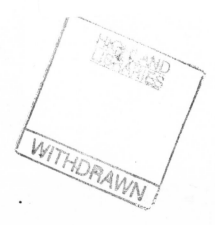

MIMI KUO-DEEMER

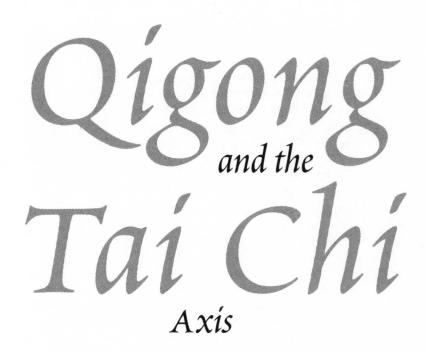

Qigong and the Tai Chi Axis

Nourishing Practices for Body, Mind and Spirit

S

First published in Great Britain in 2018 by Orion Spring
an imprint of The Orion Publishing Group Ltd
Carmelite House, 50 Victoria Embankment
London EC4Y 0DZ

An Hachette UK Company

1 3 5 7 9 10 8 6 4 2

Image on page 52 courtesy of the Wellcome Collection

Grateful acknowledgement is made for permission to reprint Chapter 9 [10 lines] from
TAO TE CHING BY LAO TZU, A NEW ENGLISH VERSION, WITH FOREWORD AND
NOTES, by STEPHEN MITCHELL. Translation copyright © 1988 by Stephen Mitchell.
Reprinted by permission of HarperCollins Publishers in the USA and Canada, and by
permission of Pan Macmillan through PLSclear in all other territories.

Every effort has been made to ensure that the information in the book
is accurate. The information in this book may not be applicable in each
individual case so it is advised that professional medical advice is obtained
for specific health matters and before changing any medication or dosage.
Neither the publisher nor author accepts any legal responsibility for any
personal injury or other damage or loss arising from the use of the
information in this book. In addition, if you are concerned about
your diet or exercise regime and wish to change them, you
should consult a health practitioner first.

A CIP catalogue record for this book is
available from the British Library.

ISBN 978 1 4091 8395 2
ISBN (Ebook) 978 1 4091 8396 9

Printed in Great Britain by CPI Group (UK) Ltd, Croydon, CR0 4YY

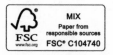

MIX
Paper from
responsible sources
FSC® C104740
www.fsc.org

www.orionbooks.co.uk

ORION
SPRING

To my parents, grandparents, ancestors,
and all who have come before me,
back to the Source that is One.

CONTENTS

PART 2

FIRE ELEMENT: NOURISHING THE HEART

PART 4
METAL ELEMENT: NOURISHING THE SPIRIT

PART 5
WATER ELEMENT: NOURISHING OUR DEEPEST WISDOM

FOREWORD

There is a word in Chinese called *yuanfen* that most directly translates as a 'fateful coincidence' – often seen when luck or destiny plays a role in bringing people together. This is how I would best describe my relationship with Mimi.

I met Mimi in 2003 when she walked into my class in Venice, California, where I was teaching my system of Sacred Energy Arts. She was like a beautiful koi fish with enormous eyes and watery movements – keen on learning more about the intersection between hatha yoga and qigong. It was very clear that she was an intelligent, focused, woman who was going to touch many people's lives. We spoke at length after class and Mimi shared with me that she had opened her own school in Beijing and would like to have me come teach there. This was the beginning of our long and fortuitous relationship.

When I think of Mimi, I think of someone as a great connector. As a Chinese American, who has lived and studied all over the world, she is a perfect ambassador to bridge the ancient teachings of the East with today's West. There is no better foundation than that of qigong.

Today's world is moving at a rapid pace – we see this in technology, population growth, and consumption. We work longer hours. We work harder. We work faster. Sometimes these demands demand too much. We become overly stressed, tired, sick, and we neglect our internal life force – our *qi*. We all have our own unique energetic signature, but unless we are willing to take the inner journey, the path is blocked, and we stray further from alignment with who we truly are. The qigong practice is the ancient Asian system of health and self-development that allows us to slow down, create s p a c e, and bring each of us back in harmony with our true Self.

Equanimity means to have a calm mind in difficult situations. This is a hallmark of qigong and tai chi practices. In Buddhism, it is described as having a mind like a clear lake. The demands of the world are not changing anytime soon, but we can change, and that change begins within.

The term *dantian* refers to our energy centre in the body. It is where an acupuncture point known as the 'Sea of Qi' resides. The journey we can take, travelling from the mind (or upper *dantian*) to the heart (or middle *dantian*) to the abdomen (or lower *dantian*), is one of the most sacred journeys we can take. This connection is the mind–body link from the cranium to the sacrum. This pathway is known in the world by many names. Qigong refers to this as the tai chi axis or zhong ding. In craniosacral circles it is known as the core link; in the Native American tradition it is the red road; in some Christian traditions it is ascension; in the yogic tradition it is the kundalini. This short physical distance of approximately three feet (one metre) is one of the most beautiful and important spiritual journeys available to us.

In this book you will find practices that can enrich your life and offer what the Chinese call 'radiant health', or 'health beyond danger'. You will be guided with Mimi's expert hands, words, wit and grace, and you will have the opportunity to enter the internal path of self-discovery – to walk the red road. May your journey bring you joy, health and freedom.

Sifu Matthew Cohen
Founder of Sacred Energy Arts

PREFACE

Qigong (pronounced 'chee-gung') is a system of Chinese medicine that has helped transform people's health and well-being for over 2500 years. Over the 15 years I have practised and taught qigong, I have seen how this ancient approach continues to benefit people, by providing tools with which to manage energy levels, regulate health and balance life.

As the popularity of qigong and tai chi extends beyond China and Asia, my aim is to reach across both cultures and present the wisdom from Chinese medicine and qigong in ways that contemporary, Western readers can appreciate and find useful. I have also chosen to focus on how we can approach qigong as a fundamentally nourishing practice for the body, mind and spirit. Although qigong certainly takes patience and perseverance, it does not require as much strength or flexibility as some systems of movement-based practices such as yoga or martial arts. As an energy-based art, the power of qigong lies in its subtle potency. Most likely, you will find that even a few minutes of qigong a day can make you feel invigorated and relaxed.

Each part in *Qigong and the Tai Chi Axis* provides an overview of seasonal themes and characteristics of the Chinese Five Elements of Wood, Fire, Earth, Metal and Water as they relate to qigong practice. My intention is to give you greater context as to why certain qigong sequences and forms are beneficial. This way, as you learn to do the forms, you can track the specific benefit that each exercise offers your physical, mental and emotional health.

In most cases, I have used the worldwide standard of Pinyin to transcribe Chinese characters. In some instances, I have used the

Wade–Giles transcription, for words such as tai chi, for example, which is consistent with how most English speakers use and reference this term. The term 'tai chi' means the point where yin and yang come into perfect balance. The tai chi axis is how we feel this balance in our bodies. The term 'tai chi chuan' (taijiquan) is different. Many people often ask me what the difference is between qigong and tai chi chuan. The easiest way to explain the distinction is that tai chi chuan is a type of qigong practice: it follows set sequences that are martially based meditative movements. These sequences have been handed down primarily by five families and lineages in China – the Yang, Wu Yi Xiang, Chen, Wu Jianquan and Hao-styled tai chi chuan. The forms in tai chi chuan are among the estimated 7000 forms of qigong found in the world today.

I hope you enjoy the stories, examples, explanations and practices that follow. More importantly, I hope you can use this book as a tool to understand why qigong can be a deeply nourishing, balancing and healing art for any age and level of fitness. With qigong's emphasis on the Five Elements, my hope is also that you may discover a way to feel a true sense of peace and belonging with the beauty, mystery and balance of nature and the universe.

Qigong and the Great Source of Wholeness

At the heart of the ancient Chinese healing art of qigong is the idea that nature is balanced and harmonious. This balance is known as the tai chi, or 'great source'. In classical Chinese texts, this source creates oneness, and it is where the natural forces of yin and yang come into equilibrium. In the body, this source is the tai chi axis. It is where we stand aligned between the earth and sky, a place and space of wholeness and health. When we orientate towards the balance of the tai chi axis through regular qigong practice, we have the potential to heal and be more fully alive.

Nourishment is also what all living creatures – plants and animals alike – seek to ensure their steady growth and health. This book is an invitation to explore the ways in which qigong can assist us, as human beings, to find this nourishment and use it to support the health of our body, mind and spirit. It offers tools to help us replenish our resources when they seem depleted or scarce, manage our energy levels and learn to make healthier choices in everyday life.

What is qigong?

Qigong is a form of energy cultivation. *Qi* in Chinese means 'life energy' and *gong* 'to cultivate'. It is considered one of the pillars of Chinese medicine, but also the basis of most Chinese martial arts, which draws its principles from Daoism and Buddhism. In both Daoism and some forms of Buddhism, qigong remains the primary means of moving and exercising the body, regulating the breath and calming the mind and/or heart on the path to spiritual awakening. It is therefore a practice that can, at once, be medicinal, martial and spiritual.

To cultivate qi, it can first be helpful to have a clearer definition of *qi*. The Chinese character for *qi* uses radicals, or drawings that combine to form words, that include steam and rice.

With these images in mind, *qi* can be understood as the product of food, fire, water and air. In the Chinese language, *qi* is part of everything. It can be used to describe the weather (*tianqi* 天氣) or one's facial coloration (*qise* 氣色) and emotional state. For example, to become angry is *sheng qi* (生氣) – which translates as 'birthing *qi*'. Daniel Keown, author of *The Spark in the Machine,* has provided a more functional definition of qi from a Western, medical perspective. He writes that qi is more than just life energy; it is the 'organising force of the body' and 'energy produced by each cell'.[1] It is in our breath, bones and blood. It animates our every movement and thought and is the energetic blueprint that gives life to all matter. When we practise qigong, we are, therefore, affecting the force that powers and structures our life.

Qigong employs a blend of active and dynamic movements, breathing, visualisation and meditation techniques aimed at culti-vating healthy qi flow through the body's organs and meridians. Qigong adheres to the principle of *xing ming shuang xiu,* or 'the body's energy, form and spirit are equally refined'. This principle assumes that the body's qi can be altered and affected: it has the potential to be clear, healthy and in balance. Because of lifestyle, trauma, injury or stress, however, qi can also become stagnant, blocked, diseased, erratic, sluggish, excessive or deficient. In acupuncture, needles are used to clear blockages in the flow of qi and support overall health through moving balanced qi into the organs and meridians. Much in the same way, qigong works to cultivate healthy qi flow where there has been disruption or imbalance. Instead of needles, however, it turns to movement, intention, visualisation and breathing techniques.

Many Westerners are just becoming familiar with qigong and its health benefits, but it has been practised in China for centuries – often under different names. The earliest forms of qigong were known as the *daoyin*, which means 'leading and guiding the qi'. *Daoyin* practices can be traced back to scrolls from 168 BCE that depicted people stretching, breathing and imitating animal movements such as the monkey, dragon, crane and bear. The movements were described as treating a range of conditions, from flatulence and rheumatism to disturbances of the nervous system and anxiety.[2]

Today, there are many branches and lineages of qigong. The estimated 7000 forms practised currently worldwide may feel overwhelming, but in some ways, knowing this can be a relief. While more martial schools of qigong, such as tai chi chuan, can be prescriptive in how forms should be executed, for me, knowing there are thousands of forms means that whenever I start thinking I'm doing something 'wrong', I consider whether I have perhaps just created a brilliant new 7001st qigong form.

Journey to the East and West

My interest in qigong began when I was living in China. Originally born in upstate New York, I grew up in the United States but began visiting China at an early age. In total, I lived in China for over 13 years between 1994 and 2009. My parents, who were Chinese immigrants, set off as students to the US from China in the 1950s, but always maintained a keen interest in Chinese politics and culture. I am grateful to them for always reminding me of the significance of China and its cultural heritage, and glad they took myself and my brothers there regularly. In fact, the first time I went to China was in 1982, when I was nine years old. Back then, just years after the Cultural Revolution, China was what many called the 'sleeping dragon': people saw its potential to rise up on the world stage, yet no one would imagine it would transform into the economic leader it is today. I feel privileged to have been witness to China's incredible transformations and changes, and to appreciate its rich traditions that have endured despite the turmoil of the last century.

For most of my time in China, I worked in journalism – first as a television journalist in 1994, and then as a freelance photographer. Starting in 2002, I also taught yoga and managed Beijing's first yoga studio. Looking back on that period of time before I began practising qigong, I probably had too many passions and not enough resources. I was burning out regularly, in an unhealthy and emotionally abusive relationship, irritable and quite fleshy – especially around my arms and belly. I often felt needy, ungrounded and overwhelmed. In short, I'm sure I wasn't much fun to be around.

Though I tried some qigong during my early years in China, it was an American practitioner, Sifu Matthew Cohen, who was my first qigong teacher. He continues to be a strong influence in my practice and teaching. Matthew studied and taught a fusion of tai chi, qigong, martial arts and yoga. On my invitation, he came to Beijing in 2004 to teach a workshop at the yoga studio I was running at the time, Yoga Yard. I'll never forget how powerful it felt when Matthew instructed me into *Wuji*, or Emptiness Stance – the qigong standing position. I felt a combination of being grounded yet energised and awake in ways that contrasted to how I felt in yoga postures. I was immediately hooked, and since then have been integrating qigong into how I practise and teach yoga.

In 2005, I began co-teaching retreats in a small village outside Beijing, near the Great Wall, called Sancha, where I rented a weekend home. The retreats were primarily led by Cameron Tukapua, a New Zealand acupuncturist who was formerly the head of the New Zealand College of Acupuncture in Christchurch. I met Cameron through one of my main yoga teachers, Donna Farhi. Cameron shared teachings about the Chinese Five Elements with our group that made a profound and lasting influence on my health, lifestyle, relationships and my general sense of my place in the world. These elements, sometimes referred to as phases, are Wood, Fire, Earth, Metal and Water. In Chinese, they are called the *wuxin*. It is believed that each element in nature relates to an organ and meridian system in the body. Alongside these teachings, Cameron also shared a powerful set practice of Five Element Qigong Forms that quickly shifted a number of long-term respiratory illnesses and digestive disorders with which I had struggled.

Cameron's teachings of the Five Elements also helped me change some of my daily routines that further support my health. I began to follow the Chinese body clock through a day, such as eating a full breakfast (the stomach is most active between 7.00 and 9.00 a.m.) and not working past 7.00 p.m. (between 7.00 and 9.00 p.m. are the heart protector hours, when we should be with our loved ones rather than with computers). In time, I began a course of self-study, reading and learning about qigong, Daoism (the underlying belief system of qigong) and Chinese medicine.

Over the years, I have learned that qigong and the Five Elements model posit balance as possible and natural for every human being. This has helped me see that certain characteristics I felt about myself – tendencies to be needy, burning out or feeling ungrounded, for example – were simply certain elemental qualities out of balance, rather than something inherently lacking in myself. I also became aware that the source of stress, tension and disease can often be traced to a lack of harmony and flow in my elemental constitution. Learning tools to work positively with these disparities in my elemental make-up has been life-changing.

Today, along with yoga and meditation, qigong, Daoism and the Chinese Five Elements play central roles in shaping my approach to living with a sense of energy, balance and well-being. This book is a presentation of the ways in which qigong and its foundations in Chinese Five Element theories in particular have offered me and my students nourishment at a deep and transformative level. Each section offers a composite of stories, information and insights shared from my studies. As I do not come from or adhere to any specific qigong lineage or tradition, this book does not present any set style or school of qigong. Instead, I offer this book as a companion to those like myself who would like to find helpful tools that can enable them to understand qigong in everyday language. It is my hope that readers of this book can learn fundamental practices while gaining insights and wisdom that support our natural capacity for nourishment of the body, mind and spirit.

Relationships between the Five Elements/Phases (*Wuxin*), Yin and Yang and the Tai Chi Axis

The Chinese model for health is based on the idea that we are a microcosm of the macrocosm. We are each comprised of organs that correspond to one of the Five Elements as well as a season. For example, Wood relates to spring and the liver and gall bladder, and Fire to summer and the organs of the heart, small intestine, pericardium and triple heater. These organ systems also link to certain times of day, colours, sounds, smells and emotions (see chart, opposite).

Together, the elements and seasons move in cycles that are part of yin and yang. Yin and yang are often described as active and receptive, light and dark, male and female. The original meaning of yin and yang, however, referred to the shady and sunny side of a mountain. Ancient Daoist and shamanic sages observed that as the morning sun rose and crossed the sky, one side of the mountain would be in sun while the other was in shade. By afternoon, the light on the mound was the opposite. This non-hierarchical idea came to reflect the notion that the world exists in a harmonious balance of opposites: if something contracts, it must first expand. In time, the idea of yin and yang was drawn as a symbol known as the *taijitu* (*tai chi tu*). In this image, the seed of yin is always within yang, and vice versa. This notion of balance is the essence of qigong and Daoism.

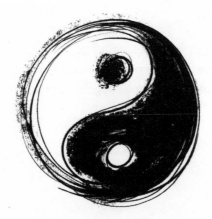

In this theory, qi is the product of seasonal and elemental movements between yin and yang. When we learn to adapt our bodies to these natural cycles, we have the potential to harmonise our qi with nature. This is the main goal of qigong: to balance our qi in the body. When this happens, we come into alignment with the yin and yang energies of our body, or the tai chi axis.

Season & Element	Direction	Organ & Meridian System	Colour	Emotion
Spring, Wood	East	Liver & gall bladder	Green	Anger
Summer, Fire	South	Heart, small intestine, pericardium & triple heater	Red	Joy
Late summer, Earth	Centre	Spleen & stomach	Yellow	Sympathy
Autumn, Metal	West	Lungs & large intestine	White	Grief
Winter, Water	North	Kidneys & urinary bladder	Blue/black	Fear

To maintain balance, there are two cycles always at work: the generative (*shen*) and controlling (*ke*).

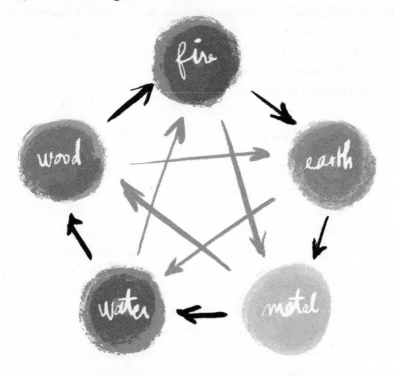

The generative cycle creates elements:

Water feeds the growth of Wood.
Wood builds Fire.
Fire burns down and its ashes create Earth.
Earth generates Metal.
Metal collects and enriches Water.

The controlling cycle restricts elements:

Water puts out Fire.
Fire softens and melts Metal.
Metal chops Wood.
Wood stabilises Earth.
Earth blocks Water's flow.

All work to create harmonious balance between yin and yang in qigong.

This framework presents a helpful perspective on physical as well as mental and emotional health. Because nature is seen to be in balance and continually cycling through the seasons, our organ systems and their corresponding qualities can also be understood to move through cycles and potentially find homeostasis, or balance. Yet because of our habits, lifestyles or other circumstances, our organs tend to feel challenged and out of balance.

Balance as a model for health

Nature's capacity for homeostasis and balance is also qigong's model for health. As human beings we are part of nature. This means that we, too, have the possibility of finding balance and alignment with the fluid cycles of change. Just as imbalance in nature may be caused by too much heat, not enough rain or insufficient nourishment in the soil, imbalances in our bodies may also be a result of excess heat, insufficient hydration or lack of nourishment to our mental and physical lives. And just as these imbalances in nature are not seen as signs that nature has failed or fallen short, we can also learn to see that our body's imbalances are not indications that we are fundamentally flawed; rather, we can see that problems arise because our elements are in or out of balance.

This important perspective gives us a way to begin having more control over our health and well-being. Qigong helps to even out the excess or deficiency of qi in the organ systems, thereby creating the conditions for healthy qi and energy flow. We can choose to work to address our body's needs by adding heat to our system if our body is too cold, or cooling the system if the body burns too hot. We can learn to soften in areas that feel rigid and stiff, or build integration and cohesion in areas that feel distant, diluted or weak. This is what acupuncturists do with needles, or herbalists with herbs.

With qigong, we use a combination of intentional, moving meditations and deep breathing to support our body's ability to maintain health. The movements are slow, steady and done so that you nourish rather than deplete the body's energy reserves. As the Han Dynasty Chinese physician Hua Tuo wrote, the 'body must have exercise, but it should never be done to the point of exhaustion.'[3] Hua

Tuo also described how this approach aids digestion, improves blood flow and prevents illnesses.

This last point is important. Qigong is a preventative medicine. It is not a cure-all or a panacea for all disease. Its focus is on supporting the body in natural ways through movements and meditations that enable our organs and meridians to function as best they can. Regular practice can reduce damage to our organs and, in some cases, reverse severe medical conditions, but this often depends on many other factors such as your genetic make-up, the severity of the disease, diet, sleep patterns and lifestyle.

The good news is that with regular practice, qigong naturally helps guide us towards adopting better habits. Through intentional movements, we begin to feel more present and sensitive to our body's needs. We pay attention to where we hold stiffness, tightness and tension, and learn to deliberately relax and soften these areas. We also consciously deepen and refine our breathing, which lets the movements become meditative. When we focus on the breath, our mind begins to calm and become steady. This can help alleviate the effect of mental stresses such as worry and anxiety. Breathing practices also begin to circulate qi. When this happens, qigong becomes more than just exercising the muscles and moving the bones. When qi effectively circulates, it means that we open the body to the uninhibited flow of qi. This nourishes our blood and helps us steady our energy levels.

When we start to feel the effects of qigong, we begin to know what it is like to be healthy, vibrant and clear. We can also sense when we feel off-kilter and imbalanced. Once we become aware of this, we have the capacity to change it. Qigong gives us the tools to see, respond and adjust to our experiences so that we can stave off the detrimental effects of fatigue, tension and stress before they become deeper problems.

Above all, qigong works to integrate the virtues of trust, integrity, wisdom and compassion into the human body and spirit. It is a practice that people of all ages and levels of experience can embrace and find beneficial. It is a simple yet profound art that has the potential to give you optimal vibrancy, happiness and health.

Guidelines for Practice

The format of this book respects the idea that qigong nourishes and balances our elemental constitutions, helping us align more closely with the flow of our natural state and the tai chi axis. This nourishment takes place at different but equally important levels of our experience. I have chosen to focus on the Five Elements and on each element's core qualities and characteristics:

Wood is an element that can help us nourish our roots and our capacity for steadiness.

Fire is an element that can help us nourish our heart and our capacity for connection, warmth and love.

Earth is an element that can help us nourish our mind and our capacity for clear, bright intention.

Metal is an element that can help us nourish our spirit and our capacity for appreciation of life.

Water is an element that can help us nourish our deepest wisdom and our capacity to connect to our essence and inborn potential.

Each section will offer general practices as well as forms from more popular qigong sequences, such as the Eight Brocades, 18 Forms, Five Animal Frolics and the Five Element Mudras and Forms. Sections will also include breathing practices, visualisations and meditations that can be subtle yet highly powerful ways to nourish and heal the body, especially when physical movement is challenging or your energy is low.

It is best to read through each section of the book first, and then begin to practise movements and meditations once you have a general understanding of the context and reasons behind practices. Many of the forms can be linked together into other sequences, which are offered in the Additional Practice Guide at the end of the book (see pages 231–5).

PRACTICALITIES FOR PRACTICE

Time of day: Active qigong is best practised in the morning, though there is no harm in doing it later in the day or in the early evening. Visualisations, breathing practices and meditations can also be done anytime, including before bedtime.

Eating and meals: Heavy meals are not advised before practising qigong, but it is always good to have a bit of food in your system before you start, especially in the mornings. The reason for this is that food starts qi production in your body and digestive system. My advice is that if you practise in the morning, drink some lemon/ginger tea, or eat a piece of fruit or toast before you start.

Where to practise: Generally, you can do qigong anywhere. Finding a clean, quiet space indoors is good, as is outside. Be sure to stay warm if you practise outside, though.

What to wear: Comfortable, loose clothing is good, but one of the freedoms of qigong is that no special kit is necessary. If practising indoors or in warm weather, you may prefer to be barefoot. However, it is advisable to never have cold feet. Therefore, shoes and/or socks should be worn to keep the feet warm, if necessary.

How to breathe: Orientate your breathing towards slow, long, even, fine and deep breaths. Let your breathing be centred around your abdominal area, or lower *dantian*. Unless you have blocked sinuses, allow your mouth to close and breathe through your nose.

The rule of thirds: If you are injured, it is advised to work to one-third of your effort level. If you are not injured, you can work to two-thirds of your effort level. Always reserve the last third of your energy and effort as a reservoir and resource. Also, if you are menstruating, you can practise these forms but reduce your effort level to half or one-third.

Resting the tongue and teeth: In most qigong practices, allow your teeth to come together without clenching. Rest the tongue on the roof of the mouth. This is believed to help join two important meridian systems in your body – the *Ren Mai* and *Du Mai*, or the main yin and yang channels of the centre-front and centre-back body.

As another general guideline for practice, we can look to a few passages from one of Daoism's central texts, the *Dao De Jing (Tao Te Ching)*, written over 2500 years ago.[4] These ancient ideas can offer some useful insights into the benefits of qigong practice for us today.

What is rooted is easy to nourish. Qigong encourages us to stay rooted, to receive sustenance and energy; otherwise, we feel ungrounded, unstable and imbalanced in our lives.

What is recent is easy to correct. Qigong enables us to become present. When we are lost in the past or stuck planning for the future, we lose our ability to be adaptable, open and responsive to the fluid, changing nature of experience.

What is brittle is easy to break. Qigong fosters suppleness and hydration in the body, like a well-watered tree's limbs. In this way, we do not snap with stiffness or dry out as quickly as we age.

What is small is easy to scatter. Qigong helps us stay open to a larger life. By teaching us that we can align ourselves with nature, which is vast, infinite and mysterious, we can remember that sometimes our small life worries and problems can often prevent us from seeing the larger picture of all the beauty, mystery and power of life moving through us at any moment in time.

Prevent trouble before it arises. As a preventative medicine, qigong suggests that if we implement strategies and align with our natural rhythms and cycles, we can stay reasonably healthy and well.

Put things in order before they exist. If you are healthy now, begin now, rather than wait until you are sick to begin practising qigong. This will ensure greater long-term health.

The giant pine tree grows from a tiny sprout. Qigong is not a solution for all illnesses and ailments. Though the effects can be immediate, and qigong can support recovery from certain conditions, the long-term benefits of qigong are most valuable when practised patiently, regularly and consistently.

The journey of a thousand miles starts from beneath your feet. Qigong asks that we begin from where we are; from where we are, we can choose to travel great distances to live a full and nourished life.

For me, these ancient jewels of wisdom speak to our capacity as human beings to live fully and awaken to our possibilities of being human. They offer us a guideline that is both practical as well as spiritual, which is part of the reason qigong can be so nourishing and healing as an art form.

Let us begin the journey from beneath our feet with Wood, and how we can nourish our roots.

PART 1

Wood Element

Nourishing Our Roots

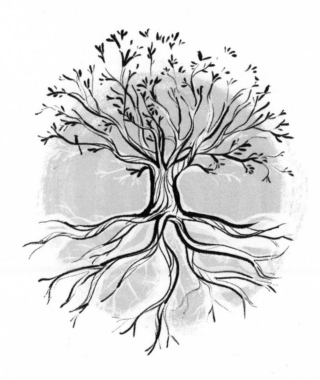

CHAPTER I

Rising Yang and the Energy of Spring

Every year in March, after the cold winter gives way to longer and warmer days, Mother Nature teases me. With increased sunlight, the appearance of flowers and slowly budding trees, I feel as though my heavy winter coat should finally come off. When a blast of Arctic-like winds suddenly blows in, however, I am reminded that March is still on the cusp of winter's end. In fact, in the northern hemisphere, March is a raucous time of year. Strong energy starts to pry us from the grip of bleak, cold days, yet we must remain flexible and patient, and slowly transition out of winter's enveloping months.

Wood in the Chinese Five Element theory

Spring and the Wood element relate to creation, beginnings, plans, initiation, optimism, power, activity and expansion. In life, all growth relies on Wood energy, be it a growing child, a muscle in our body or future plans. Wood energy is creative. Its spirit is something called the *hun*, or ethereal soul, which lives in the otherworldly landscape of our dreams and imagination. It emerges from the darkness and emptiness of winter and the Water element, to burst forward with potential and possibility.[1]

Wood's characteristic is to grow both crooked and straight. This energy complements the rising yang quality of expansion that stretches upwards and outwards. When in balance, Wood's qualities are rooted, firm and steady. From these steady roots, trees will grow with clear purpose and direction.

In the Five Element cycle, Water, which corresponds to the season of winter, feeds and nourishes Wood. Throughout the winter months, Wood's roots have absorbed nourishment in preparation for an abundant and splendid growth in spring. Wood then matures in summer. By late summer, if a plant or tree is fruit-bearing, it will deliver a healthy harvest. By autumn, growth slows down. Leaves fall off trees, returning back to the earth as compost. By winter, most trees focus their energy on resting. They produce little new growth, but instead soak up nutrients from the soil and rainwater to prepare once again for a spring bloom. This cyclical process of wood's growth, decay and rest enables some trees, such as the giant redwood and yew, to live for hundreds if not thousands of years.

Like anything in nature, however, challenges in a tree's environment can cause imbalance to wood. When there is too much water, roots will rot, and a plant may never grow. Likewise, if there is too much restriction in growth – for example, if a pot is too small for a plant's roots – the tree will likely be arrested in its development. It will be hungry for soil, but when none is available, it will feel restricted, confined and unable to absorb nourishment. If a plant grows and is never cut back, it can overreach, or branch out in too many directions. The cutting back of Wood is governed by the element Metal, which chops and directs the way in which Wood grows. This restriction stops Wood growing beyond its healthy range.

Helpful metaphors can be drawn for how we might learn from these different circumstances. Like wood, we seek healthy growth and development, but we also require the right conditions to execute our plans, visions and dreams smoothly. If we cling to circumstances and fear change, we risk feeling stuck, or end up drowning out our possibilities to grow. If we seek growth but feel limited by our circumstances, we can feel frustrated – like we're living in a pot that is too small. If we plan too many projects and branch out quickly without the rest and quiet of winter, we may burn out before any of our ideas come to fruition. We may also feel chaotic and confused without clear direction and purpose, or feel as though we have been treated unfairly.

With healthy, balanced Wood energy we experience growth as fertile ground to nurture our vision and dreams. We also have a clear sense of how these dreams can become a tenable reality. When our Wood energy is harmonious, we may feel more content and aligned with the way the universe unfolds: organically and without struggle. We may also sense a deeper trust in the Source, or wholeness of life.

For myself, having an understanding of spring and a language around the Wood element's spirit has not only helped me align more closely with the seasonal energies in nature, but it has also infused my practice of qigong with new levels of appreciation. As I practise qigong, I do so with the knowledge that the intention behind the forms is orientating me towards healthier, balanced Wood energy.

The following section offers techniques and practices to awaken and support our body's Wood element. We start this awakening process by establishing healthy roots in our physical form.

CHAPTER 2

Finding Stability and Root

In Chinese, there is an idiom that says if the roots are deep, the foundation is strong: *gen shen di gu*. In qigong and tai chi chuan, there is similar emphasis on creating deep roots, so that any movement outwards or upwards is predicated on a solid foundation.

To feel and embody this idea, we can explore the Chinese concept *chen*, which means 'to sink'. In English, the phrase 'to sink', however, does not convey a positive feeling or image. We tend to think of a sinking ship or sinking energy levels. Merriam-Webster defines the verb 'to sink' as 'go to the bottom', 'become partly buried (as in mud)', or 'to become engulfed'. It implies dropping to a lower level or even disappearing from view. Therefore, if I heard a qigong teacher tell me to 'sink' down without understanding the meaning of *chen*, I might feel a bit down or low in energy!

The principle and practice of *chen*, however, is quite the opposite of feeling buried. In Chinese, the word means to submerge, to immerse, or drop down in a deep, profound way. *Chen* is often used to help students stand and let go of rigidity or unnecessary tension. It enables them to begin finding deeper roots for a stable, nourished foundation.

If we consider the character for *chen* in Chinese, it uses the radicals for water (the three small diagonal lines on the left), a roof (the top section on the right side) and a desk (the long lines beneath the roof).

$$沉$$

These are interesting ideograms to visualise in our body. With the radical for water, *chen* invokes qualities of depth, wisdom and flowing down to the deepest places, which is what water does in nature. We are also invited to practise *chen* with the same humble offering that water gives the earth: it nourishes and supports all life, without ever asking for anything in return.

When we then add the radicals for the roof and a desk, *chen* then also suggests the image of a writer or scholar deeply immersed in their studies beneath the safety and structure of a home. In ancient China, scholars were esteemed members of society who were able to focus their knowledge and go beneath the surface of experience and share wisdom with the imperial courts. When we invoke *chen* in our bodies, we are invited to sink like the roots of a tree and go beneath the surface of experience and know it in depth. We can also begin to absorb deeper reflections and insights about how qigong can nourish our body, mind and spirit.

Standing Qigong Posture (*Zhan Zhuang*), or Emptiness Stance (*Wuji*)

The position for standing meditation is arguably the primary and most important position to learn in qigong. There are two names for the posture: one is simply called Standing Qigong Posture, or, translated more directly, Standing Post. Another name is Emptiness Stance, or *Wuji*. I will use the latter name of *Wuji* as I believe it lends useful imagery and deeper meaning to the practice.

Wuji is the stance taken before any other movement or forms begin. It aligns the body so that our feet stand firmly on the earth and our head lifts towards the heavens. In qigong and Daoist philosophy, the human body is seen as the conduit between heaven and earth; *Wuji* becomes a template through which heavenly yang and earthly yin energies can begin to flow into and through the form of our body. In this way, *Wuji* also invites us to orientate towards the movement, interplay and balance of yin and yang that is the tai chi axis.

To practise *Wuji*, we draw on the principle of nourishing our roots through *chen*. When done with sincerity and regular practice, *Wuji* creates foundations for healthy alignment and allows the body to begin circulating qi in an effective and revitalising way. As the emphasis on root in *Wuji* steadies the physical body, the mind can also become more steady, calm and focused.

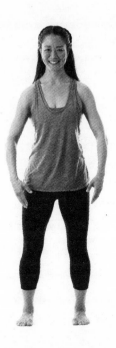

As human beings, however, having a calm mind is not always easy; the mind's tendency is to try to think its way through problems – we worry, fret or replay the past. As this happens, everything suffers: our blood pressure rises, breathing quickens and our whole system becomes strained. Qigong techniques teach us how to bypass the busy and often troubled mind by training and strengthening habits in the body, such as knowing how to find centre and root down into the earth. This way, in the face of sudden change or distress we aren't carried away. *Wuji* invites us to delve into the form of the body directly and to steady it. By learning to stand rooted, we can become anchored in a physical steadiness that then supports the mind when encountering difficult situations. In time, we can also train the body to continue to breathe deeply and enable the muscles to relax, even when we are distressed. This is because the body has built up sufficient memory and resources to help mitigate the effects of that stress.

The instructions for *Wuji* are varied across many traditions of qigong. I have compiled those that I share with students when I teach, and which have worked for me to support and nourish a sense of grounding, calm and presence in my body and mind.

When beginning, aim to practise *Wuji* for 2–3 minutes, and gradually build up to 5–10 minutes. Eventually, a seasoned practitioner can do *Wuji* for 30 minutes or longer as a standing meditation practice.

Wuji is a complex pose with detailed instructions. You may want to start with a basic understanding, and then explore the more nuanced approaches as your practice deepens.

BASIC FORM INSTRUCTIONS

1. Stand with your feet shoulder-distance wide, feet pointing straight ahead.
2. Take long, slow, even, smooth (as opposed to coarse) and deep breaths.
3. Bend your knees slightly.
4. Relax your arms by your sides, leaving a slight gap between them and the sides of your body.
5. Relax the joints of your body.
6. Allow the tailbone to descend while the crown of the head rises.
7. Actively relax your whole body as you stand – this is called *fang song*, which in Chinese translates as 'placing into relaxation'.
8. Place the tongue lightly against the roof of the mouth, behind the teeth. Let the teeth close without clenching.
9. Soften your gaze downwards, eyes open or closed.
10. Create an inward smile.
11. Remain for 3–5 minutes, working gradually up to longer periods of time.
12. To finish, transition gradually out of the pose by bending your elbows back and straightening the legs. Then relax the hands down, as though they were resting on the surface of water. Notice how you feel.

DETAILED FORM INSTRUCTIONS

As you practise *Wuji*, you may wish to integrate more detail and begin to refine the position. Upon first reading, the next set of instructions may seem like quite a lot to absorb and integrate; with practice, however, they become familiar and intuitive.

1. *Breathe long, full, even, fine and deep breaths into the lower abdomen, or the lower* dantian. *The* dantian *means cinnabar field, or the place where the elixir*

of life is ploughed, planted and harvested. Consider the lower *dantian* as the reservoir of qi in your body. It is located 7.5 cm (3 inches) beneath your navel centre. It is the primary place where qi is cultivated, refined and stored.

2. *Stand with your feet shoulder-distance wide and outer edges turned straight.* This wider base of support allows for more steadiness in your stance, and hence more ability to find stability throughout your body.

3. *Spread the toes and balance the weight on the feet evenly.* Take a moment to fan your toes. Then shift the weight forward towards the balls of your feet until you nearly lose your balance and tip forwards without doing so. Then rock back towards the heels, again almost until you lose your balance, but without doing so. Then rock forwards again, but a bit less; rock backwards again, but less. Continue to rock back and forth, each time a little bit less, until the movement becomes subtle and barely noticeable. When you reach this point, you have found even weight and balance between the front and back of the feet.

4. *Root the feet.* Begin to practise the art of *chen*, or going beneath the surface. This helps to root your feet and steady your foundation. You also allow for energy to yield down, which in turn grants pathways for a rebound of energy back up through the body. There are nine points through which you can root, and one primary pathway through which energy can rise and nourish the body.

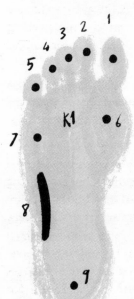

The nine points through which you root down are:

Points 1–5 pads of each toe

Point 6 ball of the big-toe mound

Point 7 outer edge of the ball of the foot

Point 8 long edge of the outer foot

Point 9 centre of the heel

The primary pathway through which you draw energy back in is the centre of the ball of the foot. This is an acupuncture point called 'Bubbling Spring', or *Yong Chuan*. It is the first point of the kidney meridian line (K1). This point is used to draw energy back up into the legs and body. If you scrunch up your toes, you will see a dimple at the centre of the ball of your foot. That is the approximate location of *Yong Chuan*.

5. *Bend the knees slightly.* As in the exercise in Step 3 of balancing the weight in your feet, you can also find a point between bent and straight with your knees, by bending them deeply and straightening them fully. Then explore bending them a bit less and straightening them a bit less a few times. When you reach a point of bending and straightening minutely, you have likely found the halfway, balanced position of neither too bent nor too straight. You can also check the position by looking down at your knees and feet. The knees should cover half your foot but not your toes.

6. *Rest the arms and relax the shoulders, arms and hands.* If you squeeze your arms against the sides of your waist, hips and legs and then release them, they will spring back into a resting position natural for your bones. Leave an acorn-sized pocket of space in your underarms. Let the arms feel soft and relaxed, the hands open and breathing. Often, the shoulders will feel tense if you lift the arms too far out. Remember to keep the shoulders down.

7. *Keep the gaze and eyes lowered.* Your eyes here can be either open or closed. One of my teachers, Sifu Matthew Cohen, suggests the eyes can remain open for a strengthening martial practice, and closed for a more healing and nourishing practice. Invite your awareness to be on the lower *dantian*, or abdomen.

8. *Invite the crown of the head to lift, but keep the chin slightly tucked.* This lets an acupuncture point known as the 100 Meeting Points open towards the heavens. The 100 Meetings, or *baihui*, is known in qigong as a 'spirit point'. It is where qi can move in and out of the body.

9. *Allow the tailbone to descend naturally towards the earth.* While some schools of qigong teach a stronger action of tucking the tailbone and tilting the pelvis, my personal experience is that too much of a posterior pelvic tilt, where the tailbone moves forward towards the front of the body, may reduce qi flow through the pelvis and spine. According to a theory offered by Sifu Matthew Cohen, the original intention of tucking the tailbone may have been to create cohesion on a horizontal plane that stabilises and protects the abdominal region. This is good for martial practice. For non-martial qigong practice, however, a more vertical stability can be

supportive of efficient qi flow through the body, particularly in the joints. My suggestion is to invite a gentle drop through the centre of the spine, all the way down through to the tailbone, which creates a balanced, neutral alignment through the pelvis and spine.

10. *Broaden the sacrum (the triangular bone between the two sides of your pelvis).* This will create widening across the lower back and kidneys without causing the pelvis to tilt. The action may be difficult to feel at first, as it can be subtle. Placing a hand on the sacrum may help you feel the sacrum widening and broadening. Widening this area will create more openness across the back of the body, which is home to the primary yang meridian, known as the *Du Mai*, or governing yang meridian in the body.

11. *Relax the whole body, including your joints.* In Chinese, this action is called *quan shen fang song*. *Quan shen* means the whole body, and *fang song* means active relaxation. *Fang* means to place, and *song* means to relax or unknot – as though untying a shoelace. Use intention to release tension and stand in an open, calm and loose manner. For the joints, in Chinese there is a saying, *guan jie song kai*. *Guan jie* means your joints, and *song kai* means to be relaxed and open. When we intentionally relax tension, especially in the joints, it permits qi to flow more efficiently through the body. This is in part because the joints in Chinese medicine are home to what are known as energy gates, or portals that open and close to help regulate the flow of qi.

12. *Create a gap and space on the surface of the skin.* This idea creates a sense of permeability and porousness in the skin, which allows the body to relax and expand. Many of the meridians are also located close to the surface of the skin; by focusing on expanding the skin, you may also support an easier flow of qi through the body.

13. *Relax the front of the torso; brighten and expand the back body along the whole spine.* The front body, from the perineum up to the abdomen, chest, throat, jaw and lower lip, is home to the primary yin meridian known as the *Ren Mai*, or conception vessel. Keeping this whole channel relaxed invites a receptivity and softness across the chest and also around the abdomen and stomach, areas where we can often hold tension. The primary yang channel, the *Du Mai*, begins at the tip of the tailbone and ascends along the centre of the spine. It continues along the back of the neck, top of the head, midline of the forehead and nose, and ends in the space between the upper lip and gums.

14. *Rest your tongue lightly on the roof of the mouth.* When you rest your tongue here, you help join the two primary channels, or meridians, in your body of the yin and yang, or *Ren* and *Du* meridians, respectively.

15. *Create an inward smile.* This is perhaps my favourite instruction. Creating a subtle, inward smile orientates our practice towards a positive rather than a grim intention. Often I see students working so hard to concentrate and focus on the details of how to execute *Wuji* that the process becomes laboured and strained. By keeping a light smile, we point our heart and mind towards a tranquil, happy state.

16. *Finish without startling spirit.* To come out of *Wuji*, move slowly so as not to startle the spirit. Begin by lifting through the centre of the body, hold one wrist with the other hand behind your back and massage the bottoms of the feet by rolling your weight across one foot and then the other. Circle on your feet 3–5 times in one direction, and then reverse and circle 3–5 times in the other direction.

Du
Mai

Ren
Mai

FINAL NOTE

While you practise, you may notice subtle, small movements and adjustments. These are normal. Rather than will the body to remain completely still, be willing to sway a little and make adjustments, the way branches or leaves might gently move in the wind, or the way your body might be moved by gentle waves. Remember: Emptiness Stance is the stance of potential and possibility. Keep the body soft so that you can be open to receive what may come in, to fill your experience.

Embrace Tree, Embracing the One
(*Cheng Bao Zhuang*)

Embrace Tree is a form that naturally continues from *Wuji*. It involves lifting the arms until they are level with the chest. Like *Wuji*, this form also has different names, both of which offer helpful imagery. For the Wood element and spring, the image of embracing a tree trunk offers a strong connection to the steadiness and rooting of a large tree. On the other hand, Embracing the One also evokes a sense that our experience is part of a wholeness and oneness of all creation.

> Like *Wuji*, you can begin practising Embrace Tree for 2–3 minutes and gradually build up to 5–30 minutes. It is not easy to keep the arms raised, though, so patient practice and a gentle increase of stamina is important, otherwise you can deplete rather than nourish the body.

FORM INSTRUCTIONS

1. Start in *Wuji*. Feel the principle of *chen*. Take slow, long, even, fine and deep breaths into your lower *dantian*.

2. From *Wuji*, slowly lift the arms and hands to the level of the chest, as though wrapping the arms around a large tree trunk.

3. Turn the palms to face slightly inwards, relaxing the shape of the fingers and hands.

4. Soften the shoulder and elbow joints. Let the elbow joints drop until they are slightly lower than the shoulders, but still in a rounded shape.

5. Keep the hands soft and receptive. Imagine they are holding something delicate, such as flower petals.

6. Emphasise the index finger while relaxing the thumb, middle, ring and little fingers.

7. To release, lower the arms back to *Wuji*, and follow *Wuji* Step 16 (page 31): finish without startling spirit.

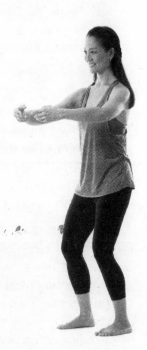

Horse Stance (*Mabu*)

In the family of standing postures, Horse Stance is among the stronger positions. It conditions the legs and increases physical and mental strength and endurance. It is also a posture from which many other sequences and forms in qigong are built, making it a good one to learn and include in daily practice.

Many of the principles in practising Horse Stance are the same as in *Wuji*: we apply the principle of *chen* to create stability and root through the feet and legs, and keep the joints of the body relaxed and open. Many of the actions through the body are also similar, such as broadening the yang channel on the back body (*Du Mai*) and relaxing the yin channel on the front body (*Ren Mai*).

> While some martial artists may endeavour to practise Horse Stance for longer periods of time, I would suggest that for nourishing the body and promoting qi flow, moderation is key. Starting with one to two minutes and working up to five is a healthy goal. Even after a few minutes, your legs will thank you when you release!

FORM INSTRUCTIONS

1. Start in *Wuji*. Take a moment to centre and breathe into your lower *dantian* using long, slow, even, fine and deep breathing.

2. Step the feet apart. The distance should be approximately 1 metre (3–4 feet). If you extend your arms to the sides, your toes should generally align beneath your wrists.

3. Turn the toes slightly out and root the feet. The toes should be positioned at an angle of 15–20 degrees. The position of the feet is to create strength, cohesion and integration. If you turn your toes too far out, you will feel unstable. Root the feet through the nine positions and draw energy up through the Bubbling Spring point described in *Wuji*, Step 4 (page 28).

4. Bend the knees. You can decide if you prefer the knees slightly bent for a milder Horse Stance (think pony ride), or if you'd prefer a deeper bend (think sitting onto a tall stallion). The knees will want to buckle in, but endeavour to keep them pointing outwards in the same direction as your second toes. This involves working your legs quite diligently, building heat, endurance and strength.

5. Open the arms to shoulder height. Keep the shoulders relaxed, elbow joints soft and hands soft. The palms can face slightly forwards and down.

6. Descend the tailbone, lift the crown of the head. Like in *Wuji*, apply these actions through the spine to create alignment and a healthy position of the pelvis (*Wuji*, Steps 9 and 10, pages 29–30).

7. Create gaps and space in the skin, relax the front and back channels of the body and create an inward smile (*Wuji*, Steps 12, 13 and 15, pages 30–31).

8. To finish, straighten the legs slowly, shift the weight to one leg and step the feet back into *Wuji*. Remember to move out of the pose as best you can without startling spirit (*Wuji*, Step 16, page 31).

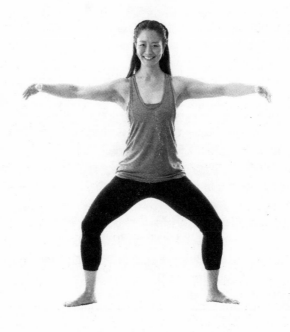

CHAPTER 3

The Resourcefulness of Trees: Flexible and Strong

In my hometown of Tucson, Arizona, my parents planted a large bamboo grove. It always puzzled me how an Asian plant like bamboo could grow in the Sonoran Desert, but I was thankful that my parents attempted and succeeded. As a child, I remember running my hands over the bamboo's clean, strong shoots, thinking, 'How can such a simple plant make me feel so much reassurance and ease?' Only later did I learn that for centuries, the Chinese have extolled the merits of bamboo.

In many classical Chinese texts, bamboo is described as a 'gentleman' among plants or like the ideal scholar: honourable and upright, supple-minded, self-assured, yet also modest. With its deep roots and ability to withstand fairly extreme changes in temperature and climate, it is also seen as a model for resourcefulness and resilience. But bamboo's good traits don't stop there! Bamboo also speaks to humility. Its centre is hollow, suggesting that it is empty like the Dao: the eternal void that is always filled with infinite possibilities; and, because it rarely flowers, it has little need for attention from creatures like butterflies and bees.

Freedom, suppleness and strength in the body: Wood's tissues of the ligaments and tendons

The element of Wood corresponds in our life cycle with early childhood and adolescence. Think about a baby putting toes in its mouth: it is as though the baby is so flexible that it doesn't have bones! Often, however, especially as we grow older, we can feel increased tightness, stiffness and anything but freedom in our bodies.

When healthy Wood manifests in our body, we feel like bamboo: strong but also responsive and pliant through our muscles, joints and limbs. When our Wood element is out of balance, however, movement can either feel stilted, brittle and stiff, or too loose and overextended due to a lack of stability. To find a healthy balance of flexibility and stability, we can start by looking at the tissues related to the Wood element – our ligaments and tendons – as well as how we think of our joints.

Perhaps contrary to most ideas, flexibility does not only mean having lean, stretchy muscles. Rather, flexibility is defined as having a healthy range of movement in your joints, as well as the ability for muscles to lengthen across a joint. Flexibility on its own, however, is not enough. In fact, as flexibility increases, chances are stability decreases, unless we counteract this. In creating balanced movement in the body, it is, therefore, best to pair the development of flexibility with an equal amount of rooting, stability and strength.

Tendons and ligaments are like the rigging ropes of a ship that allow for movement while keeping the ship's frame solid. They work to create the basic structures of stability, so that your muscles and bones can move within a safe and well-structured environment.

Tendons: The function of tendons is to connect muscles to bone. Their primary job is to modulate force as we move – in other words, they allow a muscle to generate force when we use it.

Importantly, tendons are not elastic and not meant to stretch at all. They can, however, become stronger and more stable, especially through movements that work a variety of muscle groups, such as those found in qigong. Their primary purpose is to create cohesion: they bind muscle fibres together as they attach to bones. They are made of 86 per cent collagen (in Greek, collagen means glue).

Tendons store energy during movement and allow muscles to create force. For example, whenever we walk, our Achilles tendon stores energy when the foot is released and sends that stored energy into action as we step the foot forward.

Tendon length is determined by our parents and ancestors. Tendons have not been shown to either increase or decrease in movement range, despite efforts to stretch them. This is unlike our muscles, which can be affected by intentional movement and releases. The only time a tendon's length changes is when it is injured.

Ligaments: The function of ligaments is to connect bones to bones. Like tendons, our ligament make-up is also determined by genetic predisposition; they are made of strong, collagen fibres; and there is very little evidence to show that they either increase or decrease in response to our actions, unless via injury.

Ligaments, however, are partially flexible. There are two types of ligaments: white and yellow. White ligamental tissue is not meant to stretch – it stabilises and holds bones together. Yellow ligamental tissue can stretch to a degree and return to its original shape. However, because very few blood vessels circulate through ligaments (blood carries nourishment through the body and deposits it in damaged cells), healing from a torn ligament can be very difficult and slow.

Joints and synovial fluid: Unless we continually move, stretch and hydrate our bodies, particularly in the muscles and joints, we begin to harden and dry out. Qigong can help slow this process down and mitigate the effects of joint deterioration by creating balanced movement in the joints and muscles. The slow, fluid movements performed in qigong also help increase the flow of qi as well as synovial fluid. Synovial fluid is the key to preventing friction between the joints. It helps absorb shock, protects the joint spaces and also supplies vital nutrient and waste transportation within the cartilage. By moving with qigong's slow, circular movements, you can help the body secrete this fluid into the joint cavity and deter or reduce inflammation or deterioration that can arise from conditions such as arthritis.

We work with exercises such as joint releases to prevent brittleness and increase qi flow. With regular practice, we can maintain our body's flexibility, and perhaps enjoy a healthy range of movement in our bodies through youth as well as our later years.

Wood and resilient mental and emotional states

In addition to supporting a balance of stability and suppleness in the body, the Wood element also teaches us that trees can be good role models for our mental and emotional states. Unlike many of us, trees meet challenges to their growth by finding ways around an obstacle. When we make plans and they fall apart or change, however, our first response is often to either give up or become angry. Both of these reactions generally cause tension. Instead of stiffening, tensing or becoming obstinate when situations fail or don't go according to plan, we can draw on the steadiness of our roots and exercise the flexibility, adaptability and resourcefulness of trees and the Wood element to find ways around our problems.

Here are some qigong practices to connect us to the flexibility, strength and resourcefulness of trees.

Joint Opening (*Song Kai Guan Jie*)

In Chinese medicine, qi can be balanced and healthy, but also stale, stuck, deficient or excessive. It moves through meridians and energy gates, many of which are located in the joints. When the joints are blocked, it causes the qi to stagnate, leading to pain, stiffness and disease. Over time, this imbalance can cause arthritis or lead to an overall lack of nourishment in the body. Excessive qi in the joints can occur when the energy gates are too full. This can manifest as inflammation and agitation.

These joint-opening exercises help create the conditions for balanced qi flow through our energy gates. They can be done in the morning or evening, as a gentle practice to revitalise and mobilise the body. They are based on a set of classical warm-ups.

Like all qigong active practices, remember to keep the range of movements moderate rather than extreme in range.

FORM INSTRUCTIONS

1. **Neck rolls.** Start in *Wuji*, taking a few long, slow, even, fine and deep breaths. Then rest the hands on the lower *dantian*, left hand over right for women, right over left for men. (This position based on gender is a guideline drawn from the concept that the left hand represents yin, or female, and the right yang, or male. As gender is far more fluid in today's cultural lexicon, I advise students to place whichever hand feels most natural on top.) Bring the chin towards the chest, allowing the back of the neck to release. Then inhale and gently bring the head towards the right shoulder; exhale and bring the chin back to the chest. Inhale and bring the head towards the left shoulder; exhale and bring the chin back to the chest. Continue moving the head and neck side to side. If there is no injury or trauma to the neck, you can begin rolling the head further back and around, creating circles. Do this 3–7 times, and then release the head back to centre.

2. **Shoulder rolls.** From neck rolls, begin to roll the shoulders forwards and up on the inhale, back and down on the exhale. Imagine there are four points – down, forward, up and back – that you roll through each time. Complete 5–7 rolls, then reverse direction and do another 5–7, inhaling as you roll the shoulders back and up, exhaling forwards and down. Release.

3. **Wrist releases.** Interlace the hands in front of the chest and begin to circle the hands and wrists in one direction 5–9 times, then reverse and repeat, circling in the other direction 5–7 times. This is very good for the wrists as well as the finger joints.

4. **Opening and closing the gates.** From shoulder rolls, bring the arms into a cactus shape: elbows bent at 90 degrees. This movement is for flexion and extension of the spinal joints. On the inhale, bend the elbows back – opening the gates. Keep the lower back safe by emphasising the elbows bending back rather than the lower back bending back. This will open the upper chest and upper back. Then exhale and extend your arms forward. At the same time, turn your arms inwards so the backs of the hands face each other. This is closing the gates. Bend the knees and extend the arms from the sides of your waist. The back should extend straight like a tabletop. Continue and repeat – opening the gates as you inhale, closing the gates as you exhale – 3–5 times, ending with closing the gates. From here, release by lifting the chest and crown of the head up towards the sky, allowing the arms to ripple back down to the sides of the legs.

5. **Arm swings for health**. This movement is for rotation in the spinal joints and muscles. Keeping the feet and knees steady, begin to let the arms swing, wrapping the arms around the front and back of the belly and waist. Swing the arms for 2–5 minutes.

6. **Side bends.** From arm swings, root the right foot into the earth as you inhale the right arm up towards the sky. Then exhale and begin to laterally extend the arm from the right foot, hip, shoulder, elbow, wrist and fingers to the left. You should feel a good release through the whole right side of the body. Remain in the side bend for 3–5 breaths, then release with an exhale. Repeat on the left side, and then release the arms down and stand back in *Wuji*. Notice and observe the sensations in the body.

7. **Hip circles.** From *Wuji*, bring the hands to the hips and begin to circle the hips gently and slowly in one direction. The circular movement and action is fairly straightforward, but you can also create more awareness and subtlety by focusing on the shift of weight in your feet as you circle from one foot across to the other. You can also pay closer attention to the movement of the tops of the leg bones, or femur heads, in the round hip joint, which is located nearer to the groin creases. Circle in one direction 7–9 times, then reverse and circle in the other direction 7–9 times. Release by lowering the arms down to the sides of the legs.

8. **Knee circles.** Step the feet and knees together. Create what is called the Tiger's Mouth with your hands: an L-shape where your thumb is at a right angle to the other four fingers. Bend the knees, gently hug the inner knees together and place the Tiger's Mouth on the tops of your kneecaps, or meniscus, and then bend the knees. Circle the knees 5–7 times, with the hands stabilising the tops of the kneecaps and the inner knees still snugly together. Reverse and change direction, and then release to standing.

9. **Ankle and foot releases.** Step the feet back apart into *Wuji*. While breathing steadily, shift the weight onto your right leg and point the left toes forward. Inhale and flex the foot, bringing the heel to the earth; exhale and point the foot, bringing the toes to the earth. Repeat 7–9 times, then change legs. Finish by standing in *Wuji*.

Pulsing/Harmonising the Qi (*Qi Shi Tiao Xi*)

Pulsing is the first form in the Tai Chi Qigong 18 Forms sequence as well as a common warm-up used in qigong.[2] Following the joint releases described above, pulsing can create strength, rootedness and resilience in the body and mind. It increases stamina and balances flexibility and strength. It is also a good practice to help deepen the breath, calm the mind and settle the liver qi. When the liver qi becomes blocked or imbalanced, it can lead to feelings of frustration. Because pulsing asks us to move with steadiness and patience, we can learn to create a sense of fluid, steady composure and ease when facing agitation or restlessness.

You can do 5–9 rounds of pulsing or even more, depending on how you feel each day.

FORM INSTRUCTIONS

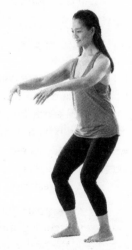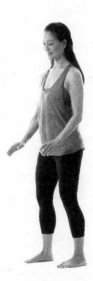

1. Stand in *Wuji*, with the feet about hip-distance wide, knees soft, arms relaxed down by the sides of the body.

2. As you inhale, lower the hips back and draw the tailbone down. The arms float forwards in front of the chest. Lift the arms more from the head of the arm bone and shoulder socket than from the hands. Let the hips draw back more than the knees bend forward. Keep the knees as stationary as possible, so that they do not bend too far forwards or move too far back towards straight. Also keep the chest soft, open and upright.

3. As you exhale, the crown of the head lifts up and the hands release down. The feet also root down to help the crown of the head lift. Remember to keep the knees bent and in the same position, so that the hips rise more than the knees.

4. Continue and repeat 5–9 rounds, keeping the hands, fingers and joints relaxed.

Rolling Ball (*Ding Bu Dao Jian Gong*)

This is another practice from the Tai Chi Qigong 18 Forms. This form can be of excellent service to stiff shoulders. It also conditions the lower back and brings qi flow to the gall bladder and liver, the two organs associated with the Wood element. When healthy and balanced, these organs help to brighten the eyes.

> The form mimics how we might throw an overhand ball. Rather than it being thrown, however, the action is to roll the ball forwards and backwards from behind the ear, creating a circular movement that conditions the shoulder joint as well as the muscles around it.

FORM INSTRUCTIONS

1. Start in *Wuji*, taking long, slow, even, fine and deep breaths. Inhale and bring your hands up to the level of the chest. Fully breathe out.

2. Inhale and extend one hand forward as the other hand reaches back behind the head, as though rolling a ball from behind the ear.

3. Exhale and draw the two hands towards each other in front of the chest.

4. As they pass each other in front of the chest, inhale and change the arms – one hand forward, one hand back. Exhale, both hands towards centre. The hands continually switch – one hand draws forward and the opposite hand draws back. It is beneficial to practise with soft, relaxed hands. Also aim to draw on inner strength to move the hands apart. This inner strength can help prevent the hands from becoming rigid or stiff as they move. You might imagine a sticky substance between them that you can stretch, such as treacle or toffee. As you move, keep the shoulders relaxed and turn from the waist. This will strengthen and mobilise the shoulders and also condition the lower back, liver, gall bladder and kidneys.

5. Repeat 6–9 times. Then, bring both hands towards the chest centre before lowering them down. Release back to *Wuji*.

6. Finish with a practice known as the Closing Form for Peaceful Qi (see page 61): Inhale and gather healthy flexibility, suppleness and resourcefulness with your hands as they reach out to the sides and then overhead. Then turn the palms to face the earth, middle fingers pointing towards each other. Begin to lower the hands down in front of your face, chest and torso, and fill with the qualities you have gathered. At the same time, clear out any rigidity and tightness, leaving your body feeling adaptable and open.

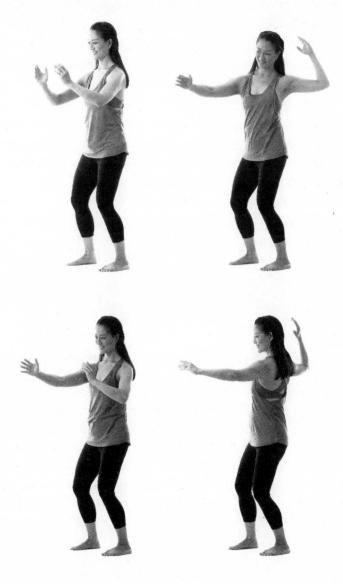

CHAPTER 4

Wood's Organs:
The Liver and Gall Bladder

In Chinese medicine and qigong, organs work in a pair that creates the balance of yin and yang. In the Wood phase, the liver is the yin organ and the gall bladder the yang. In acupuncture and qigong, focus is usually given to supporting the yin organs. This is because these organs, called the *zang*, are responsible for creating and storing qi and blood. If there is sufficient blood or qi in these organs, then it is like having a fully charged battery that can power life.

The yin, or *zang*, organs in the body are the liver, heart, pericardium, spleen, lungs and kidneys. Yang organs are called *fu*. They primarily transmit and digest food and waste. The yang, or *fu*, organs are the gall bladder, small intestine, triple heater, large intestine and urinary bladder. As we explore the organs, it is helpful to understand that each pair completes a yin/yang balance that supports the balance and wholeness of the tai chi axis. Yang organs are non-essential for life. For example, people can have their gall bladder removed, which is considered a yang organ, and still live. You cannot, however, live without your liver, which is a yin organ. Yin organs govern and store blood. When we practise qigong, we tend to focus more on the yin organ, which nourishes the blood stored in these organs. Yang organs then help move and circulate this life energy through the body.

The Liver

In Western medicine, the liver performs everything from regulating chemical levels in the body to releasing substances that make blood clots. It produces bile, a sticky substance that aids digestion, as well as cholesterol, which is needed to make hormones such as oestrogen, progesterone, testosterone and adrenal hormones. The liver also produces the proteins needed to stop bleeding, and stores sugars. These sugars are broken down and released into the bloodstream when glucose is needed – for example, when our sugar levels fall low, such as in the middle of the night, when we are asleep, hopefully, and have not eaten for at least a few hours.

The role of the liver in Chinese medicine and qigong is primarily to store blood. Since ancient times, classical Chinese texts have described how blood is the physical expression of our sense of self, or our essence, and where our mind resides.[3] Blood has also been thought of as energy that fills every cell. Like our essence (*jing*) and spirit, blood shapes, nourishes and determines who we are. It also governs smooth flow and helps us take life – and its unpredictable ebbs and flows – in our stride. This allows our emotions and energies to adapt to the many changes we face on cellular levels as well as in general life experience. In addition, the job of the liver is to ensure that our blood, water and emotions are

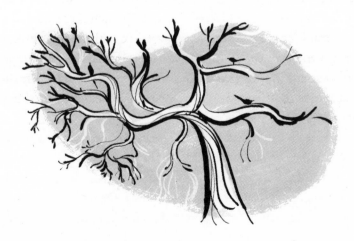

not congested or clogged, but can move efficiently around the body. It does this by absorbing indigestible components of our food and drink, such as toxins from alcohol, coffee, pesticides and chemicals in our food, and excreting them as harmless substances into the bloodstream or bile. Emotionally, the liver absorbs and releases anger. For example, when we face situations that we cannot control, a healthy liver enables us to take this in, but then also lets us express our anger in a healthy way, without blaming ourselves or others, or becoming irate. When the liver is dysfunctional, we can become moody, angry and challenged by life's sudden grim turns.

For Chinese medicine, the liver also opens into the eyes. In this way, it relates to the way trees grow in clear directions and with purpose. In fact, the inside of the liver looks remarkably like a branching tree without its leaves. It is the organ related to our plans, goals and dreams. Some equate the organ to a master architect that is responsible for designing the rhythm of our days or how we move forward in our lives. When in balance, the liver helps us be resourceful and creative in our efforts to actualise our life plans. When our liver is imbalanced and dysfunctional, this can cause our decision-making abilities to suffer, or lack inner vision. We may also experience health problems related to sleep, digestion and vision, such as insomnia, irregular bowel movements and eye diseases.

The Gall Bladder

The gall bladder is a small, pear-shaped organ located behind and underneath the liver. Its primary job in the body is to store bile. Bile breaks down fats and lets us absorb vitamins like A, D, E and K and utilise calcium. Interestingly, bile is also an antioxidant that removes toxins from the liver and expels them through our stools.

The gall bladder rules judgements and decision-making. If the liver is the master architect, the gall bladder is the engineer. It implements the liver's plans and visions. If it is overburdened and the architect pushes it too far, the gall bladder becomes imbalanced. On a physiological level, this happens when the liver produces too much bile. With excess bile, our body's toxicity may increase and our gall bladder may not be able to process and release all of it successfully. On a mental and emotional level, we may also feel a need to lash out. This is mostly due to too much energy in the gall bladder, and is the origin for sayings such as that person 'has a lot of gall'. When we say this, it implies that someone is being rude, impatient or expresses themselves too boldly or brazenly – a sign of a gall bladder imbalance.

THE LIVER AND GALL BLADDER MERIDIANS

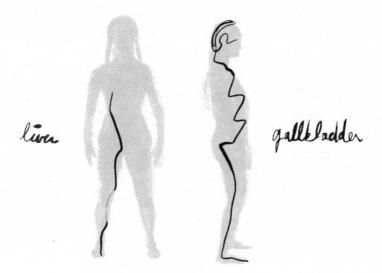

liver   gallbladder

LIVER

In the organ/element correlations, each organ also has a certain time of day when it is most active. For the liver, this time is 1.00–3.00 a.m. Ideally, this is a time of day when we are sleeping and in deep-dream states. It is also when the liver releases the most insulin to support the body's need for glucose.[4]

The liver meridian begins at the big toe, runs along the top of the foot to the inner leg, up to the genitals, to the side of the trunk and ends on the chest, beneath the nipple.

GALL BLADDER

The gall bladder's most active hours are 11.00 p.m.–1.00 a.m. It's best to be deep in sleep during these hours. Interestingly, this is when there is the highest incidence of violence and murders in the world.

The gall bladder meridian runs from the outer edge of the eye, around the upper ear to the back of the ear, zigzags up the head and down to the base of the skull, base of the neck and armpit, and then zigzags to breast, side ribs, belly, buttocks and down the side of the leg, ending at the outer little toe.

Qigong Practices for the Liver and Gall Bladder

Qigong practices for the liver and gall bladder can help us mitigate the tendency towards anger and acting out in inappropriate or destructive ways. They also support our body's ability to create, store and regulate blood, while fostering clear vision and realisation of goals, and leading us there through kind intentions.

Here are three practices that are among my favourites for the liver and gall bladder organs and meridians.

Five Element Wood Practice

I first learned this form in the mountains outside Beijing, where I rented a home for nearly 10 years. The acupuncturist and teacher Cameron Tukapua taught this to me along with the other Five Element Qigong Forms that are offered in this book. The results of practising these forms have been transformative on many levels. They work primarily with tracing the meridian lines of the liver organ with the hands, but also bring in visuals such as embracing a tree and nourishing the liver and gall bladder.

FORM INSTRUCTIONS

1. Start in *Wuji*, taking long, slow, even, fine and deep breaths. Then step the feet together.

2. Inhale, step the left foot out, knees bent, and begin to trace the fingers up from the inner, medial side of the front thighs up to the space beneath your ribs. This is part of your liver meridian line. Use gentle pressure on the skin as you trace.

3. Exhale, bend the knees and press the heels of your hands gently into the torso beneath your ribs, massaging as you press down towards the abdomen. On the right side are the liver and gall bladder organs.

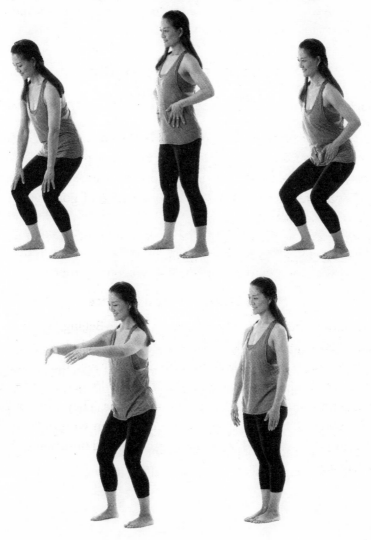

4. Inhale, straighten your knees slightly and bring your arms forward into Embrace Tree. Imagine your arms wrapping around an invisible, smooth, large tree trunk. You can also visualise your body rising like a solid, rooted tree with flexible, strong branches.

5. Exhale, step the left foot in to the right, releasing the arms and hands down.

6. Repeat Steps 2–5, stepping out with the right foot. Repeat this series 5–9 times each side.

7. After you complete 5–9 cycles, step back out into *Wuji* for the Closing Form for Peaceful Qi (see page 61). Begin to extend the two hands to the sides and overhead. As you do this, gather the qualities of Wood in balance: clear direction, growth, vision and kind intention. Turn your palms to face the earth, moving the hands down in front of the face, chest and belly. Fill with these qualities. In the wake of these qualities filling your body, you can also clear out misdirected frustration, irritation or anger – aspects of Wood that may arise when the element is out of balance.

8. To finish, bring the hands to rest on the lower *dantian*. Pause. Notice how the body feels.

Opening the Bow to Let the Arrow Fly
(*Zuo You Kai Gong Si She Diao*)

This form is traditionally the fifth form of the Eight Silk Brocades, a classical qigong sequence of forms. These were originally part of 'leading and guiding the qi' practices known as the *daoyin*, or Daoist yoga. As silk brocades, they suggest soft, silken movement.

Many of these practices address more than one organ system and element. This practice, which uses archery as its main inspiration, supports the liver and its sense organ of the eye. When you cultivate good vision, your gaze is lucid and precise. Out of balance, you may feel like your aim is fuzzy or misdirected. This practice also helps condition the heart and lungs. It builds stamina in our lower legs and creates suppleness and strength in the upper chest and mid-back – areas where our circulatory and respiratory systems are located. It also strengthens our arms and hands, where the meridians of the heart and Fire organs, as well as the lungs and Metal-associated organs, are located.

You can do this practice on its own, as part of this sequence of liver and gall bladder exercises, or as part of the Eight Silk Brocades (see Additional Practice Guide, page 233).

FORM INSTRUCTIONS

1. Start in *Wuji*, taking long, slow, even, fine and deep breaths.

2. Step the feet wider into Horse Stance, bending the knees and letting them track the toes. Open the inner legs and lengthen.

3. As you breathe in, start to straighten the legs (or keep them bent for stronger practice) and draw the hands in, forearms together.

4. As you breathe out, bend the knees again and bring the backs of the hands towards each other, making soft fists. Take a moment here, breathing, feeling steady, strong in the legs, with the intention for clear, healthy vision.

5. Inhale, straighten the legs slightly.

6. Exhale, bend the knees and pull an imaginary bow open. One hand makes an L shape, thumb and index fingers open, other fingers folded in. The other hand pulls away, as if stringing an arrow into the bow.

7. Inhale, retract back into centre, hands in soft fists.

8. Exhale, change the hands, pulling back with one hand as you look at the other; index and thumb extended so they become the gauge for your bow.

9. Continue, repeating for 5–9 rounds. You inhale and release, exhale and draw open the bow, aiming the arrow with clear vision and direction.

10. To finish, step the feet closer and release the arms and hands to *Wuji*. Notice how you feel.

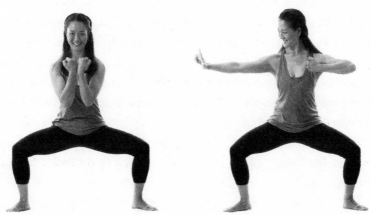

DEER FORMS

Like the Eight Silk Brocades, the Five Animal Frolics are among some of the oldest, classical qigong forms of the *daoyin*. These exercises were depicted on scrolls dating back to 168 BCE. A number of them were named as the Bear, Monkey and Bird. Later, around the 3rd century CE, a famous Chinese doctor named Hua Tuo created a systematised set of practices he described as the 'Five Animal Frolics'. The sequence included movements based on the tiger, deer, bear, monkey and bird. Hua Tuo nearly lived to be 100 years old. He is famous for being one of China's earliest surgeons, but also known for his principle of using herbs and exercise as preventative medicine. Today, he is considered to be the father of Chinese medicine.[5]

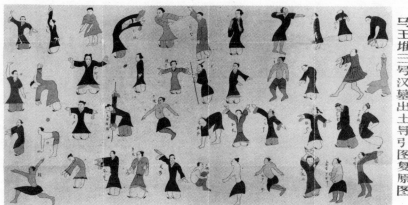

马王堆三号汉墓出土导引图复原图

The Deer Frolics correspond to the energy and movement of spring. Many of the forms include techniques that help strengthen the tendons through resistance and isometric contraction around joints. They also follow coiling patterns through the spine that suggest the movements in spring, which are to spiral upwards and outwards. The deer represents grace, sexual vitality and spirit.

There are different variations of the Deer Frolics. I have chosen two – a male and female deer – that are among my favourites. The Male and Female Deer Forms improve flexibility, strength and grace. The Male Deer gives emphasis to strengthening and lengthening the tendons; the

Female Deer flexibility through the hips and legs. You can do these on their own, as part of this sequence following the Opening the Bow exercise above, or as part of the Five Animal Frolics.

To practise the forms, visualise a light, playful quality and calm, open spirit.

INSTRUCTIONS FOR MALE DEER

1. Start in *Wuji*, taking long, slow, even, fine and deep breaths.

2. Inhale and make hooves with two hands by bringing your fingertips together and placing them at the level of the lower *dantian*.

3. Exhale, step your right heel out in front and slightly to the right. Simultaneously move your 'hooves' to the left.

4. Inhale, shift 70 per cent of your weight to the front right foot, bend the knee and lower the toes. Simultaneously make deer antlers with your hands and circle them overhead.

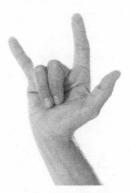

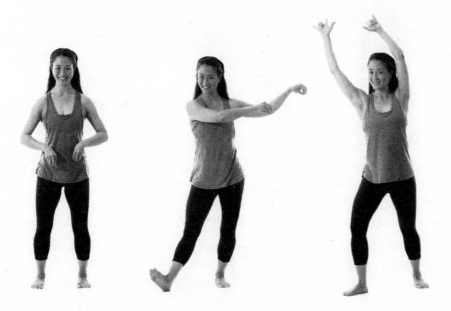

5. Exhale, keep the left arm overhead while you bring the right arm lower to the level of your waist. Simultaneously turn to the right, turning your whole pelvis, spine and chest to begin facing as far back as is comfortable. Keep the chest and torso upright.

6. Inhale, turn your 'antlers' of the hands to also face the space behind you.

7. Exhale, look back at your back left heel.

8. Inhale, sweep the arms to the right and overhead, beginning to change your antlers back to hooves.

9. Exhale and untwist, bring the arms and hands back to the left and down to the lower *dantian*. Simultaneously shift your weight to the back leg and step the front foot back to *Wuji*. Remember to keep your hands in hoof shapes.

10. Repeat Steps 2–9, stepping out with the left heel and moving your 'hooves' to the right. Repeat each side for 3–5 rounds.

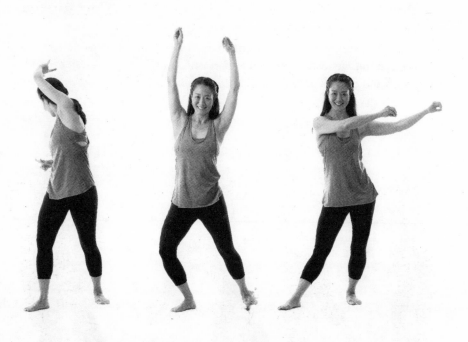

INSTRUCTIONS FOR FEMALE DEER

1. Start in *Wuji*, taking long, slow, even, fine and deep breaths.

2. Inhale and make hooves with two hands by bringing your fingertips together and placing them at the level of the lower *dantian*.

3. Exhale, bring the hooves up to make female antlers near the top sides of your head (the female antlers are like soft fists). Simultaneously shift the weight to your left leg, bend the knee and draw the weight of the hips back. Also place the right toes pointed forwards, lightly touching the ground.

4. Continue in this position, and take five long, slow, deep breaths. Keep your eyes focused softly, as though you could see very clearly and authentically into the space around you. The weight on the back leg strengthens the back thigh and foot, increasing stamina and strength.

5. Inhale, shift the weight forward, lowering the right heel.

6. Exhale, turn your back left foot outwards to 45 degrees.

7. Inhale and begin to turn towards the left, bending the back left knee. Keep the front right leg straight.

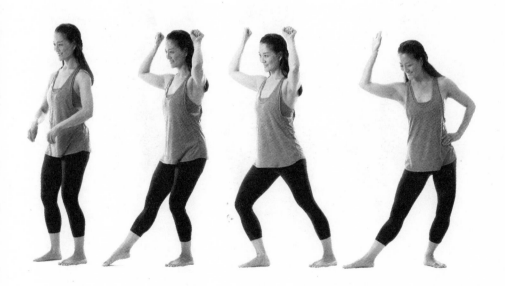

8. Exhale, release your left hand to the left hip and your right hand towards the front right shin or foot. Remember to keep the front right leg straight as you fold, and imagine you could touch your own hoof.

9. Inhale and begin to rise up, turning back to face the front with your hands as female deer antlers.

10. Exhale, step forward and release the antlers out to the sides and back down to the starting position of *Wuji*.

11. Repeat Steps 2–10 on the second side.

12. To finish, stand in *Wuji* and end with one round of the Closing Form for Peaceful Qi: use the intention of clearing out anything that feels fuzzy or uncertain, like doubt. Gather with the hands reaching to the sides and up overhead. Then turn the palms towards the earth, gradually lowering them down in front of the face, chest and belly. As they move down, fill the body with a sense of clear purpose, deep intention, insight and clarity. Notice how you feel.

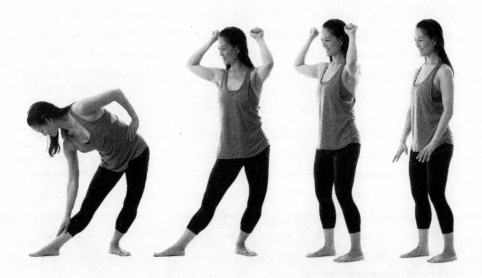

CHAPTER 5

Wood's Spirit and Emotion

When in balance, Wood's emotion manifests as anger with clear purpose – such as anger at social injustice or unfair treatment. It is a normal, healthy emotion in Chinese medicine and qigong. With healthy Wood, we assert ourselves and stand up for what we believe to be just. We are also guided by clear decisions that guide us to assert our authority and power in positive ways. When excessive and out of balance, however, Wood's anger can be like a raging, howling wind. This can manifest as being overly assertive, inflexible, angry and aggressive. It can also lead to doubt or a stubborn clinging to mistakes or bad plans. When Wood's anger is deficient, we may abandon our plans too easily and cave in to others' opinions. This can lead to a feeling of meekness. When Wood's anger is in balance, we begin to see that we can bend with the winds rather than hold on to the way things should be.

In Chinese, there are two characters for anger. One is *nu*, which is comprised of the radicals that mean 'slave' on the top (made of the radicals for a woman on the left, and the radical for a hand on the right) and the radical for the 'heart/mind' on the bottom. This combination illustrates the emotions of a woman beneath the hand of a slave master, with a general sense of tension. It can also suggest the anger of a heart that is enslaved, or the tension of the heart when in a subservient position. This type of anger is confining, and can lead to bitterness or fierce retaliation – like an explosion against authority.

Another Chinese meaning for anger is a phrase, *sheng qi*, which means 'to become angry'. A direct translation, however, is 'to give birth to qi'. This type of anger has the potential to be directed rather than explode or simmer as resentment and bitterness. We can notice when the feeling of anger boils up and respond to it by choosing to direct it in a responsible and positive way. When we do this, we have the potential to enjoy the gifts of Wood, which are transforming anger into creative ideas, or directing it towards a fair, righteous and just vision for ourselves and others.

生氣

Indeed, the moral spirit of Wood is benevolence and kind action. This kindness supports justice and actions that are guided by love, which is akin to the work of Dr Martin Luther King Jr. In the Han Dynasty book, *Discourses on a Balanced View*, Wang Chong describes how each element is linked to different ethical traits. For Wood, he writes that the ethic is humaneness, or *ren*.[6] In Confucian beliefs, *ren* is a virtuous quality felt when one performs something authentic and kind. It refers to a core human trait to love others and create positive interactions.[7] In Chinese philosophy, medicine and qigong, this moral virtue is the product of healthy, clear, balanced Wood.

Here are a few practices that can help us orientate our emotions of anger towards kindness, or *ren*.

Punching with an Angry Gaze to Increase Strength (*Wo Quan Nu Mu Zheng Li Qi*)

This practice is the most external of the Eight Brocades and 18 Forms. It is aimed at increasing strength as well as vitality. It is said to help prevent arthritis, reduce stress and improve concentration. It is also good for the liver, and helps rid the body of unhelpful, unskilful anger, while improving inner strength and clear direction. Remember: Healthy anger can help create positive change; inappropriate anger can lead to aggression or violence. Absence of anger can also manifest as lack of assertiveness, or an inability to stand against injustice and cruelty.

You can do this practice as a series for Wood's emotion, or as part of the Eight Brocades or 18 Forms.

FORM INSTRUCTIONS

1. Start in *Wuji*, taking long, slow, even, fine and deep breaths.
2. Keep the eyes focused and the gaze sharp.
3. Inhale, step the feet slightly wider than shoulder distance, knees bent.
4. Make soft fists with both hands at the level of the waist.
5. Inhale, and on the exhale, punch forward with one fist, turning it as it extends.
6. Inhale, retract that fist. Exhale, punch with the other fist.
7. Continue, breathing and alternating the fists punching forwards.
8. To finish, stand in *Wuji* and observe how you feel.

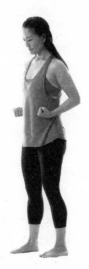
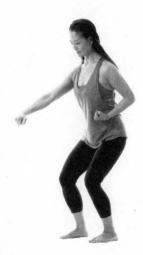

Qigong Spiralling Hands Mudra

This movement draws on the spiralling movements of plant growth. It uses a hand shape that has symbolic meaning. In Sanskrit, these symbolic hand gestures are called *mudras*. This mudra for the Wood element helps calm and steady the mind, allowing it to respond to situations rather than lash out and react. The movement of the hands follows the patterns of trees and plants, which always grow crooked as well as straight. When practising this moving mudra meditation, tap into a feeling of smooth, steady movement and of spiralling energy in and out of the torso and arms.

You can do this practice as part of this series on Wood's emotion, or as part of the Five Element Mudra practices (see Additional Practice Guide, page 232).

FORM INSTRUCTIONS

1. Start in *Wuji*, taking long, slow, even, fine and deep breaths.
2. Exhale, turn the right-hand palm to the left in front of the chest, fingers towards centre and up towards the sky. At the same time, slide the left hand down towards the earth, palm facing left.

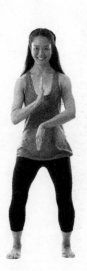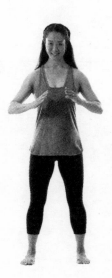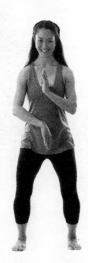

3. Inhale while beginning to draw the hands back towards centre.

4. Exhale, change the hands: left hand up, right hand down in a spiralling pattern.

5. Inhale, begin to switch and exhale, change.

6. Repeat Steps 2–5 and 7–9 times.

7. Finish by slowly lowering the hands, and stand back into *Wuji*. Notice how the body, heart and mind feel.

Closing Form for Peaceful Qi
(*An Zhang Ping Qi*)

This clearing, gathering, sealing practice for Wood is a simple, classical qigong practice that uses intention and simple movements to affect the emotions and movement of qi through the body.

FORM INSTRUCTIONS

1. Start in *Wuji*, taking long, slow, even, fine and deep breaths.

2. Breathe naturally and with awareness in the *dantian*. Continue this *dantian* breathing throughout the following movements.

3. Turn the palms out and begin to move them slowly and deliberately to the sides and overhead. As you do this, gather any unnecessary feelings of irritation, annoyance and frustration. These are mild types of anger that can manifest in our experience.

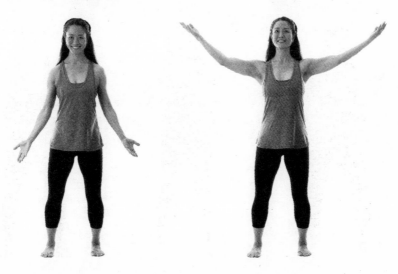

4. Once the hands are overhead, turn the palms to face the earth, middle fingers pointing towards each other, elbows bent.

5. Slowly and deliberately begin to lower the hands down in front of your face, neck, chest and belly. Use the intention to clear out any unnecessary feelings of irritation, annoyance and frustration.

6. Repeat Steps 3–5 with a different intention: gather qualities of consideration, friendliness and kindness. Fill into the space you have cleared.

7. Gather all you have filled: consideration, friendliness and kindness. Seal this into your roots to help you nourish balanced Wood in the form of your body.

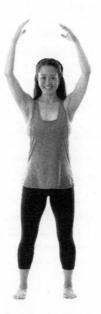 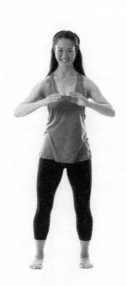

FINAL NOTE

Once you have finished all three movements, remain in *Wuji* for a few breaths and absorb the way you feel. You can complete this by placing your palms on the lower *dantian* and noticing how you feel.

PART 2

Fire Element

Nourishing the Heart

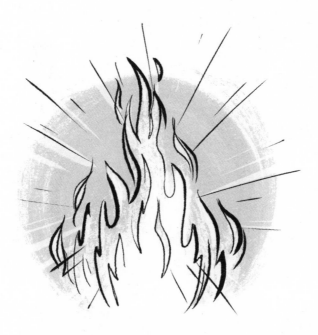

CHAPTER 6

Maximum Yang:
Fire and the Heat of Summer

If spring's growth sends forth blossoms, then summer's fire matures this growth. Summer relates to ripening, fulfilment and the maximum of yang energy. Many of us have positive associations with this season: beaches, holidays and barbecues. When this quality of maximum yang is in balance, we can feel creative, expansive, joyous and full of energy. Yet no one can sustain constant productivity, joy and enthusiasm. When we overextend ourselves – which I have often done in my life – we can feel depleted, like we want to do nothing other than curl up in a ball. When this happens, qigong suggests we start to give our heart more attention and care. The heart is the primary organ of Fire. When in balance, we open to the qualities of expansion associated with summer and the Fire element. When out of balance, however, we can feel restless, anxious or withdrawn. In the following sections, we will look at qigong practices that can fuel a balanced Fire element and nourish our heart.

Fire in the Chinese Five Element theory

In our life cycle, Fire correlates to the years we mature into adults. As our physical height and stature steadies, our growth is directed towards deepening and enriching our relationship with ourselves and with others. In our Fire years, we ideally build our communities of friends or family, meet a partner and discern what it is that we most love to do or makes us most happy.

Openness is also an important quality of Fire. With balanced Fire, we learn to respond skilfully to those who give us love and warmth and open up to qualities of love. We live in a world, however, where love is overly associated with romance. This makes discovering the beauty of other types of love, such as love between friends or a deepening love for nature, elusive. It is universally given love that begins to kindle warmth, ease and what Chinese medicine and qigong refer to as the 'divine spirit', or *shen*. *Shen* animates our life, bringing qualities of laughter and joy to the way we live. A closer look at *shen* can be found in Chapter 10.

Openness and love are not always available to us, though, and this is understandable. When we have been hurt, we close down to love and to Fire's sources of warmth. This is natural and, thankfully, in qigong and Chinese medicine any tendency to close down is not viewed as a permanent condition, but rather as a deficiency that can be met by nourishing and supporting our body's innate need for Fire. Since learning about qigong and Chinese medicine, I have noticed that on the numerous occasions when I have been devastated and feel like my heart has shattered into a thousand pieces, remembering this perspective has helped me regain my bearings and start to open up once more to all that life offers. Through qigong and other practices such as acupuncture or herbs, we can gradually rekindle our Fire and our capacity for love. This is done by providing the right conditions and patiently nourishing our constitutional Fire back to a healthy, strong flame.

It is important to remember, however, that Fire – like all the elements – is a powerful force that can be positive as well as destructive. Fire can scorch and burn, but also awaken potential for growth and possibility. It is a tool that our species has learned to use and apply to our evolutionary advantage and development, but we know that it must be contained so as not to burn down all that we build, such as our livelihoods, communities and homes. Fire needs boundaries to help it be directed towards good use.

In qigong and Chinese medicine, we want to build and maintain a steadily burning flame that keeps our body and heart warm. This will enable us to experience an inner radiance that allows us to feel more open and relaxed. For example, with good Fire, we may be inclined to spend more time with people we like and naturally wish to be social with them, and we may develop more caring and compassionate relationships with ourselves and with others. So, how do we begin this process? First by recognising and realigning with Fire's natural inclination to move towards an extreme, and then by reining it gently in. We can also nourish the heart with skills and practices that let it be content and at ease.

CHAPTER 7

The Supreme Sovereign

What is the heart? Physiologically, the heart is the muscular organ about the size of your fist that sits between the lungs, slightly left of the sternum. As part of our body's cardiovascular system, the heart's job is to tirelessly pump blood through our body each day. This work of beating and pumping has been unfolding since the eighteenth day of being conceived in our mother's womb. In the world of metaphor, our heart has also been on adventures. We have been broken-hearted, whole-hearted, faint-hearted or even eaten our hearts out! The range of the heart's experience is as vast as a cloudless sky. It holds the sublime and profound. It experiences excitement, laughter and joy, and yet it can also feel as cold as stone.

In Chinese medicine and qigong, the heart is considered the sun and supreme sovereign of the body. It is one of four Fire organs in the body (we will explore the other three organs in Chapter 9). It is the emperor or empress that governs and rules over the empire of not only the physical but also our individual psychological and spiritual identities. It is where we feel life pulse through us; the moment it stops, we die. The ancient Daoists believed that when our heart's spirit is fully refined, we become the Oneness that is the tai chi axis, and the eternal Dao.[1]

In China, the sovereign is considered the emperor who governs and oversees the well-being of the land. The emperor, or sovereign, was also the Son of Heaven, and given a mandate to rule. His role was to maintain peace and harmony by governing with intelligence and an enlightened mind. If the sovereign was not enlightened or intelligent, he would lose his mandate and make everyone in the kingdom suffer.

By living according to the rules of the Dao, understood to be The Way that governs nature and the cosmos, the Son of Heaven would ensure that Heaven's virtues and love were manifest on Earth.

As supreme sovereign, the heart's role in Chinese medicine and qigong is the same. Its primary domain is overseeing the kingdom of our body. When in balance, it is radiant like the sun and shines its love and generosity in all directions. A nourished, full heart allows us to appreciate beauty in the world – whether that be in our friendships or through art, music, nature or poetry. Our heart also inspires and compels us to live fully and use our energies towards creative goals. Its longing for sincerity, authenticity and connection makes us feel nurtured and fulfilled.

Yet when we have been hurt and our hearts ache or break, our ability to be inspired, feel connection or seek relationships with others diminishes. Indeed, sometimes heartbreak causes our own hearts to stop beating. In Western medicine there is a condition called 'broken heart syndrome', where people who have lost their loved ones die from heart attacks within a day of their bereavement.[2] For these people, the loss is too much of a burden to bear. As the organ that 'takes on the burden of the Ten Thousand Beings,'[3] our heart can be strong, but also vulnerable and full of despair.

How, then, do we work with such a complex organ in qigong? We must begin by understanding that when we meet with the heart in qigong, we are meeting it on three levels: the physical, mental and spiritual. All of these levels benefit from practices that can provide our heart with the care it requires.

1. **Physical**: At the physical level, qigong moves qi through the body via the blood vessels to extend nourishment throughout your system, reaching every cell. The smooth, circular movements used in qigong support our cardiovascular system by increasing the overall volume of blood flow to the hands, feet and brain. Often, practitioners will notice that their hands and feet become warmer – areas of the body that are furthest from the heart. This is due to an increase in blood circulation and flow. Physically, our heart also feeds itself the most oxygen-rich supply of blood first. Taking the time to do practices

like qigong that work on our circulation can be a way to extend care to ourselves before we begin to care for others.

2. **Mental**: Stress on the heart tends to create overstimulation and anxiety, so qigong's aim is to use mental focus and intention to quiet the mind. Many qigong forms are like moving meditations that help us regulate our sensory inputs and stress triggers that challenge the heart. Practices that specifically focus on the heart organ also support its function as the supreme sovereign. Ideally, we want our sovereign strong yet calm, brave yet also kind and generous. By quieting our mind, we encourage our heart to respond to life in steady and trusting ways.

3. **Spiritual**: Qigong practices that focus on the heart also begin to awaken the divine spirit, or *shen*. Movements, meditations, visualisations and breathing practices focused on the heart begin to create a spark of inspiration that awakens and brightens our *shen*. As this happens, our connection to insight, inspiration and compassion grows deeper. See Chapter 10 for more on the *shen*.

THE HEART MERIDIAN

The heart's most active hours are 11.00 a.m.–1.00 p.m. For most countries, this is when the sun sits highest in the sky. During these hours, it is a good idea to avoid heavy exercise or heavy manual labour. In fact, studies have shown that greater damage happens to the heart for people who have heart attacks in the morning versus other periods of the day.[4]

The heart meridian begins internally at the organ of the heart, and then emerges towards the surface, just under the skin, at the upper inner arm. It then travels down the inner arm through to the wrist, palm and little finger. It ends at the inner edge of the pinkie nail.

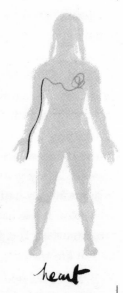

heart

When the heart is healthy and thriving, four main qualities begin to flourish that are paradigms of a good leader: openness, strength, clarity and compassion. When the heart is balanced, it is light and expansive. This is the natural and innate state of the heart in Chinese medicine and qigong. Often, however, we lose touch with these qualities as a result of stress, fear and doubt. Qigong helps remind us that we are capable of knowing and abiding in this natural state. It also offers practices to support this remembering.

The mind/heart that holds paradox

These days, our minds tend to guide and direct our decision-making. Though many of us wish we could trust and live by our hearts, usually the heart is considered less trustworthy: it is irrational and emotional, especially if at odds with the head. In Chinese, however, the word for heart, *xin,* is often interchangeable with the word for mind. For example, in Chinese the word for a psychologist is *xinli daifu,* or a doctor for the inner mind/heart. This idea of having a mind/heart gives greater breadth and depth to the heart's possible capacities to hold experience and care for it.

If we extend our decision-making capacities to something like a mind/heart, we may see that the heart is home to far greater resources. If we only use our mind to make decisions, we may easily feel frustrated and anxious. This is because many questions rarely offer straightforward answers: Does he love me? Will my child be happy? Will I age gracefully? When faced with questions of this nature, our mind understandably frets and tightens. This is because it likes to feel in control and have clear answers; it naturally seeks logical solutions to the things that bring uncertainty, confusion or pain. If someone is angry at us, we want to know why and what we may have done wrong. When a fatality happens or someone close to us dies, we want to know why, how and what can be done about it. Our efforts to understand are important and should not be overlooked. Yet sometimes our need to find answers prevents us from being caring towards the complexity of any experience. The heart, however, is different. It is stronger. In fact, it possesses a generous capacity to be with uncertainty and accept duality. If I read the papers, my heart breaks when reading about the violence and anger unfolding in the world. Yet, as I sit here and breathe right now, I can also feel immensely grateful for the warmth of my body, steadiness of my breath and blueness of the sky.

As the emperor or empress of your body, the heart has been given the mandate to govern. Its strength is that it can face difficulty while staying open to all that is beautiful, mysterious and sublime. Our heart can feel happy and sad at the same time, and know that despite whatever hardship may be unfolding, things are still OK. Unlike the mind, the heart is equipped to hold paradox. When the mind seeks the certainty of answers and cannot find them, rather than continue to let the mind tighten and feel overwhelmed by not having an answer, drop down into the domain of your heart. There you will find a deep resource. Remember that as your supreme sovereign, your heart's innate resilience is always there to help you find the strength and compassion to be OK with harder emotions such as jealousy, pain, confusion and sadness.

Qigong Practices for the Heart

There are many practices in qigong for Fire that revolve around the heart, and for good reason. When it suffers, the rest of our body suffers. These are four simple qigong practices that can help us nourish and reconnect to an open, strong, clear and compassionate heart. Though some of these forms are from specific qigong routines and can be done as part of those set forms, I have chosen to create these as a standalone set of forms to support the heart.

Parting Clouds

The sequence starts with Parting Clouds, which metaphorically clears clouds away from the sun of the body: the heart. It increases mobility in the wrists, fingers and hands, and can be a wonderful antidote to computer or other repetitive work. It can also help soothe arthritic pain in the joints of the hands and create healthy synovial flow through the joints of all the fingers and wrists.

FORM INSTRUCTIONS

1. Stand in *Wuji*, taking a few centring breaths that feel long, slow, even, fine and deep.

2. Draw your hands to the sides, level to the chest. Exhale.

3. Inhale while bringing the hands in towards the chest. As they approach each other, keep your palms facing the sky before letting the fingers begin to spiral one-by-one towards each other. This creates a full circular rotation through your wrists. Roll them as much in sequential order as you can: little finger, ring, middle, index and thumb.

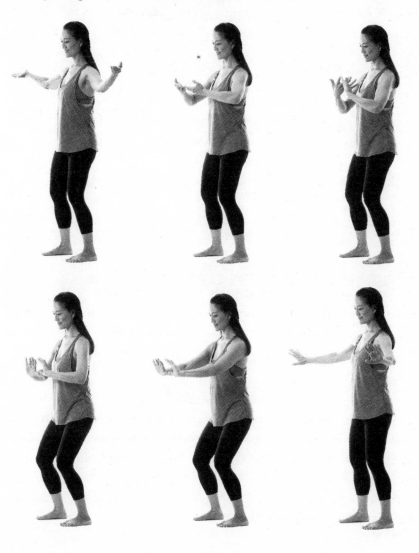

4. Exhale, move the palms away from your chest and out to the side. This is the action of parting clouds.

5. Repeat 5–7 times, inhale, moving the hands and arms out to the sides; exhale, drawing the hands in, roll the fingers and part the clouds from in front of the chest and heart.

6. To finish, release the arms back down by the sides into *Wuji*, noticing the effect of the practice.

Opening the Chest
(*Kai Kuo Xiong Huai*)

With a clear sky around the heart, you can then begin to expand the heart through Opening the Chest. This form is the second of the Tai Chi Qigong 18 Forms. It conditions the heart and lungs, stimulating and dredging the associated meridians of these organs that run through our arms and fingers. This form is also particularly good for hypertension and high blood pressure, as it encourages smooth blood flow through the cardiovascular and respiratory systems.

Though this form can be done as part of the 18 Forms or on its own, I like performing this form after Parting Clouds. For me, once the clouds have moved away from the chest and heart area, I imagine the area around my shoulders and chest can expand, and feel more radiant and bright. When this area is more relaxed and open, we can feel more spacious and relaxed in our hearts. This may help us be more receptive and awake to everything around us, enabling us to develop a more authentic and optimistic outlook on life.

FORM INSTRUCTIONS

1. From *Wuji*, inhale the arms forward, palms facing each other, and open to the sides, opening the chest. Be careful not to extend the arms too far back. You should be able to see them in your peripheral vision. As your arms extend forward and then out, the crown of the head also rises. As the arms extend to the sides, keep the shoulders relaxed, away from your ears. Also keep the hands as soft as they can be without being limp. The elbows stay slightly bent throughout the movement.

2. Exhale, bring the arms back down to the sides, softening and bending the knees.

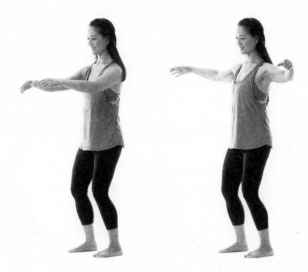

3. Continue and repeat 5–7 times. Remember to keep the arms and hands soft and elbows slightly bent.

4. To finish, release the arms back down to the sides, and stand in *Wuji*, noticing the quality of breath and space in the area of the arms, chest and shoulders.

Five Element Fire Practice

This Five Element qigong practice focuses on the Fire meridians for the heart, small intestine, pericardium and triple heater. It gently stimulates some of the Fire meridians such as the small intestine (see page 92), which starts on the outer nail of the little finger, as well as the triple burner that runs along the top of the hand. The gesture of lifting the hands towards the sky also moves the energy upward, which is similar to Fire's expansive yang qualities, and feeds and nourishes the heart by sliding the hands through the centre of the body.

FORM INSTRUCTIONS

1. Start in *Wuji*, taking long, slow, even, fine and deep breaths. Then step the feet together.

2. Inhale and step out hip-distance wide with your left foot. Simultaneously join the outer edges of the little fingers together and lift the arms overhead, as though you could raise the light of the sun towards the sky.

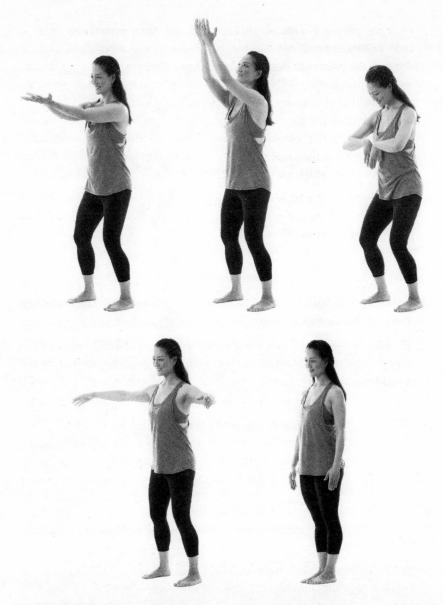

3. Exhale and turn the fingertips towards the earth, backs of the hands rolling together and descending down the centre line of the torso, as though you could fill sunlight into your heart centre.

4. Inhale the arms out to the sides, like a parasol.

5. Exhale, the left foot steps back in next to the right.

6. Inhale, stepping the right foot out. Repeat Steps 2–5.

7. After completing 5–7 rounds on each side, step the feet shoulder-distance apart one more time, into *Wuji* for the Closing Form for Peaceful Qi. Inhale and turn the palms out to gather the qualities of Fire in balance: gentleness, ease and tranquillity. Begin to lift the hands to the side and overhead, imagining them filled with these qualities. Turn the palms down to face the earth and move the hands down gradually in front of your face, chest and belly. As you do this, use your hands to fill your body with the qualities of Fire in balance, at the same time clearing out tendencies to feel agitated or overstimulated, which are qualities of the heart when out of balance.

8. To finish, place the hands on the lower *dantian*. Remain in *Wuji* for a few breaths, feeling the generous capacity of the heart when in balance. Observe the qualities of the practice.

Hands to Heart

This sequence finishes with Hands to Heart, which brings energy from the two directions to the energetic heart centre, nourishing and replenishing energy and the capacity for the heart to reign fully over the body in generous, caring ways. It invites us to bring nourishment from our hands, which are considered the messengers of the heart, to be placed on the heart as a gift. It is one of my favourite qigong practices for the heart, and one that I find many students appreciate and quickly feel benefit from in their day. This is in part because the practice is simple, powerful and profound. Rarely do we care for our own heart. Through this movement, however, we can feel both the healing and deeply nourishing effects of gifting our hands to our own hearts.

FORM INSTRUCTIONS

1. Stand in *Wuji*, breathing long, slow, even, fine and deep breaths.

2. Inhale, extend the palms out to the sides, hands open to receive nourishment and resources from all directions. You can also focus on drawing in energy from the centres of each palm. These are acupuncture points known as Working Palace, or *Laogong*, and are considered spirit points through which you can draw energy into the body, as well as give it out to others or the world.

3. Exhale, lower the chin and simultaneously bend the elbows and bring the hands in to the chest.

4. Complete your exhale by resting one hand over the other onto the centre of the chest. Traditionally, you can rest the left hand over right for women, and right over left for men. Let the palms stay open, fingers relaxed, elbows soft and placed by the ribs.

5. Take a few long, deep breaths with your palms on the chest, nourishing this area and the heart organ. This is also known as the area of the middle *dantian*, or middle energy centre, where we cultivate qi and begin to awaken our divine spirit, *shen*.

6. Then, inhale and lift the chin, drawing the hands back to the sides. Repeat Steps 2–5 three times.

7. You may wish on each movement to focus on the act of nourishment. As your hands draw in, consider what supports and sustains your heart; bring this in through the hands to rest on your heart, as though you could feed it to your heart.

8. Finish by gently releasing the arms and hands. Bring the chin back to being level with the ground. Stand once more in *Wuji*, observing the effects of practising Hands to Heart on your body, mind and spirit.

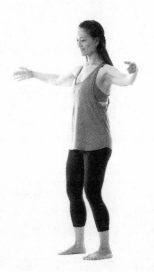
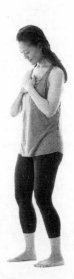

CHAPTER 8

A Calm and Tranquil Heart

Cities like London and Beijing offer excitement on tap. For 22 years, I have lived in one or other of these two capitals. I now live in the British countryside, but still, I love the pulse and rhythm of people, history and creativity that animates city life. The buzz from a thriving culture sparks my Fire energy's hunger for stimulation. Yet I also know that too much of this stimulation overloads my senses and wears me down. I doubt I am alone. Most people I know who live in London or other big cities experience burnout. Many feel distracted. Almost everyone I know works hard and feels stressed. The majority seek more peace, ease and quiet – qualities that in Chinese medicine and qigong nurture the heart – but find them difficult to attain.

What can qigong teach us about enjoyment minus the burnout? A lot. Most importantly, whether you live in a large city, small town or village, qigong helps us understand that the optimal condition for the heart is not to push, demand and drive our physical and mental states to the point where we become depleted. Instead, we can understand that wholeness and balance is not a boring, hermit-like state, but rather one that lets us embrace life and respond to its richness fully. Working hard and feeling calm are not mutually exclusive. In qigong, to be calm and tranquil means to be relaxed, composed and pleasant. Rather than collapsing when we've pushed too far, a peaceful heart can decide when and how we choose to work or rest. This ability begins by cultivating a heart that is tranquil and calm.

Finding time for rest, or creating a calm, tranquil environment, however, presents challenges for most of us. Perhaps we have children who demand constant attention, or a job that is stressful and unsatisfying. Maybe our relationships are strained, or we live in an area that is polluted, noisy and distracting. All of these situations can cause stress and imbalance in our heart. When this imbalance arises, the rest of the body struggles.

According to the World Health Organization, heart disease remains the leading cause of death in the world. Most Western doctors cite poor diet, smoking and a lack of exercise as the primary reasons for this trend. While Chinese medicine and qigong would concur, they would also point to disturbance of heart qi that results from too much excitement and general excess as an equally significant factor behind this trend.[5]

Excessive heart qi means too much heat, or Fire, which leaves us feeing physically parched and brittle. Conditions such as high blood pressure and hypertension may result. Mentally, we may be prone to feeling agitated, aggressive, scattered, or as though everything we do is frenzied or in excess. People with too much heart Fire may also laugh inappropriately. For example, this might be someone who snickers or laughs at someone else's heartbreak or pain. Excessive heart qi can lead to conditions such as anxiety, insomnia, agitation or manic mood swings.

Often, when we have excess qi, it can burn up so quickly that it puts the fire out. This can tip a person quickly to a state of deficiency, where there is not enough heart qi produced. If this is true, we can feel cold, especially in our hands and feet, and suffer from a general lack of circulation. This can lead to low blood pressure, fatigue or general sluggishness. We may also feel withdrawn and find it hard to laugh in situations that are genuinely funny. Mentally, we may feel isolated, and emotionally, we can feel afraid, sad or depressed.

Ideally, the heart and Fire energy in the body is balanced: not so strong that it singes and sears our body, like a blazing hot summer sun – nor too weak, like a fire's embers that are about to go out. When our heart qi is balanced, it is luminous and bright. It rules as it should – the benevolent sovereign of the kingdom or queendom of our body. But if the heart is overburdened, overextended and anxious, the ability to rule is undermined, and the empire suffers.

How do we best support our heart in its role as supreme sovereign? We can begin by practising specific qigong forms that can invite the heart to feel unburdened, light and spacious.

Four Qigong Practices to Balance Heart Qi

Qigong forms nourish our heart with movements and intentions that focus on improving the circulatory system as well as stimulating flow through the Fire meridians. Some of the forms, such as the Crane practice from the Five Animal Frolics and Separating Clouds, promote a feeling of levity and lightness which can help lift the spirits. Others, such as the Eight Brocades practice of Nod the Head and Wag the Tail to Calm Heart Fire, work specifically to calm and steady the heart qi.

Nod the Head and Wag the Tail to Calm Heart Fire
(*Yao Tou Bai Wei Qu Xin Huo*)

This is the fifth form of the Eight Silk Brocades. It works to reduce excessive heart qi as well as replenish any deficiency, should there be one. It also builds strength in the legs and feet, flexibility in the spine, and brings a sense of peace and calm to the mind.

> You can do this form as part of this sequence, on its own, or as part of the Eight Silk Brocades.

FORM INSTRUCTIONS

1. Stand in *Wuji*, taking a few centring breaths that feel long, slow, even, fine and deep.

2. Step the feet wider apart into Horse Stance. The knees will turn out and bend; toes turn out about 45 degrees. Place the hands onto the tops of the thighs, near the knees.

3. Inhale. As you exhale, turn towards your right leg, sliding the head and chest towards the thigh, through centre, and then over to the left leg.

4. Inhale and come all the way back up, lifting the torso upright but still keeping your hands on your thighs.

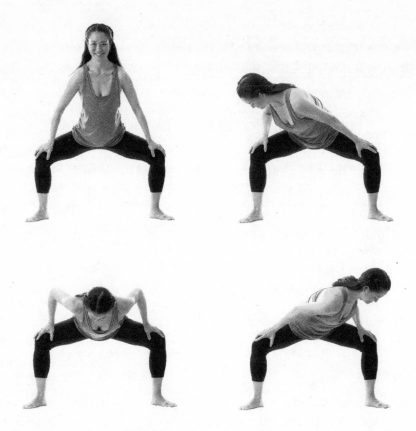

5. Exhale and extend down towards the left leg, back through centre, and come up again from the right side. This completes one full cycle.

6. Continue, repeating Steps 3–5 to help calm your heart Fire. Complete 5–7 rounds.

7. To finish, step the feet back into *Wuji*, releasing the arms. You can end this brocade by gathering a sense of calm, balanced heart Fire in your hands. Lift your hands to the sides, filled with this calm, tranquil qi. Then turn your hands, palms facing down, and fill this into the body. At the same time, you can imagine clearing out agitation and overstimulation – things that tend to offset the calm.

CRANE FORMS

Symbolising longevity, purity, fidelity and peace, the Crane forms in qigong invite our spirits to feel so light and lifted they could soar. When practising, use a calm, steady rhythm. This will condition the circulatory and respiratory systems, but also create a moving meditation, which helps quiet the mind and steady the heart. Some systems of the Five Animal Frolics attribute the crane to Metal and the lungs, but in the Frolics I have learned and practised, the crane relates to maximum yang, Fire and summer. In his book, *The Way of Qigong*, Kenneth Cohen describes the crane as 'light, relaxed and excellent for the heart and to keep the body cool in summer'.[6]

Flying Crane

This form of Crane uses the crane's beak – a position for the hand that stimulates many of the Fire, as well as Metal, meridians that run through the fingers, hands and arms. It also improves flexibility through the ankles, strengthens the legs and is therapeutic for the hands and wrists. If you spend time working at a desk or computer, Crane can be an excellent practice to help relieve the effects of carpal tunnel or repetitive stress injury (RSI).

You can do these forms on their own, as part of this Crane sequence, or with the other Animal Frolics.

FORM INSTRUCTIONS

1. Stand in *Wuji*, taking a few centring breaths that feel long, slow, even, fine and deep.

2. Bring the feet together. Then turn the toes out to 45 degrees, keeping the heels together – like a ballerina's first position. Keep your gaze steady and focused.

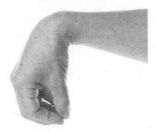

3. With each hand, touch your fingertips to your thumb. This is the hand position of the crane's beak.

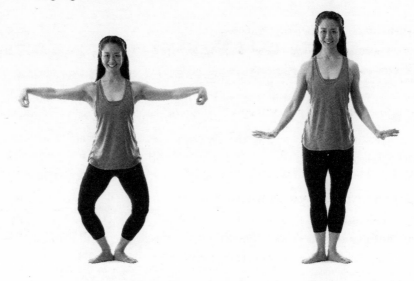

4. Inhale, bend the knees slightly out, lowering your centre. Simultaneously draw your arms to the sides, curling all the fingertips towards your wrist. The hands should lift to shoulder height. As much as possible, lift less from the wrists and more from the armpits, as though the underside of your arms could expand. This will help prevent your shoulders from lifting and tensing.

5. Exhale and begin to straighten your legs while you release the arms and fingers down by your legs.

6. Repeat 7–9 times.

7. You can finish here, stepping back out to *Wuji*, or continue to the next Crane form described below.

Red-Headed Crane Delights in Seeing its Mate

As suggested by its name, this is one of the more playful forms of qigong. Red-crowned cranes, named after the patch of red skin on their crown that glows bright red during mating season, mate for life. When they find their better half, they can dance, whoop and honk at each other for hours. This form speaks to the playfulness of the heart when in balance, but also to the feeling of happiness when finding your true love. The Chinese believe that when we find the right partner, we can enjoy a smoother path through life.

FORM INSTRUCTIONS

1. Start from the end of Flying Crane, arms relaxed by your sides, heels together and feet turned out at 45 degrees. Continue to breathe with slow, long, even, fine and deep breaths.

2. Inhale, bend your knees and lower your hips towards a squat. Imagine your hands could begin to wrap around a large nest in front of your knees.

3. Keep inhaling as you shift your weight onto your right leg and foot. Begin to stand on your right leg, floating your left knee up to your chest. As an alternative, you can also rest the left toes on the ground.

4. In one smooth movement and on one inhalation, begin to stand, crossing your arms in front of your chest and then lifting them overhead before lowering them to shoulder height.

5. Exhale, lower the arms to the sides and rest your left heel down, back to the starting position.

6. Repeat Steps 2–5, with the weight on the left foot.

7. Repeat each side 7–9 times, creating a rhythmic dance that demonstrates an enthusiastic response to seeing your mate!

8. Finish by stepping the feet out into *Wuji*, letting your breath and pulse steady. Notice how the body feels.

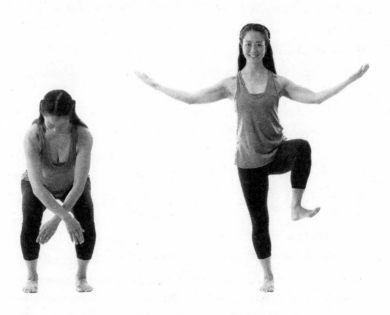

Separating Clouds
(*Lun Bi Fen Lun*)

Like Parting Clouds, Separating Clouds invites us to use our hands to move clouds, which is an unlikely feat. However, the image and intention are evocative. With Separating Clouds, the arms move overhead and to the sides, as though you could part clouds from above your head. The image of separating clouds creates a softness as well as fluidity to movement, which can engender the calm, tranquil states preferred by the heart. By separating clouds, we are also invited to rise up into the atmosphere. This can help us feel spacious, light and free.

This form is part of the Tai Chi Qigong 18 Forms, but it also has the more generic name of Cross Hands from tai chi chuan and qigong. It is beneficial to the heart and lungs, and helps open the shoulders and refresh the mind by increasing the flow of oxygen through the brain. You can do this as part of this Crane sequence, on its own, or as part of the 18 Forms.

> Keep the eyes open or closed, but focused internally to the area of the lower *dantian*. Keep the movements gradual and smooth.

FORM INSTRUCTIONS

1. Stand in *Wuji*, taking a few centring breaths that feel long, slow, even, fine and deep.

2. Inhale and cross your hands and arms in front of your chest, lifting them overhead. As they lift, imagine you are taking off a T-shirt.

3. Exhale, turn the palms to face out and fingertips up, and gradually lower the arms out to the sides and back down. As your arms come down, imagine you can separate soft clouds and let golden sunlight radiate through the sky.

4. Continue, repeating Steps 2–3, 6–9 times.

5. Release the arms to the sides, standing in *Wuji*.

6. Finish with one round of the Closing Form for Peaceful Qi (see page 61), by extending the hands to the side, gathering nourishment to your heart. Lift the hands overhead, and then turn the palms to face the earth,

middle fingers pointing towards each other. Slowly and gradually, lower the hands down in front of the face, chest and belly, filling with nourishment. Simultaneously clear what crowds and burdens the heart. When you finish, place your hands stacked on the lower *dantian*. Notice how you feel. Observe how the body feels.

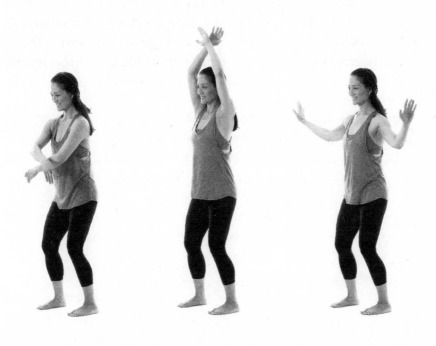

CHAPTER 9

The Heart's Three Helpers

In addition to my qigong practice, I have a daily practice of yoga and mindfulness meditation. With mindfulness meditation, one of the primary focuses is tracking my thoughts and emotions as they arise in my experience. For example, as I sit in meditation, I may start thinking of a person who troubles me, or with whom I have a difficult, unresolved relationship. If left to my habits, I would trip my way into stories about this person and become ensnared by questions of why, how and what now? Letting these stories play out invariably causes me mental and physical anguish.

Typically, the stories in my head obfuscate feelings happening in my body. If I use mindfulness, however, which best translates as 'embodied presence', I can ask, 'Where am I feeling this in my body?' In most cases, I feel troubling people or scenarios in my belly. My belly is my gut – or small intestine. In Chinese medicine and qigong, this is where efforts to separate out pure from impure are happening. As we shall see, it has a special relationship to the heart.

When situations like this arise in meditation, I am often reminded that my whole body is involved in any experience, even though I might initially only be aware of something in my head. Armed with this awareness, I begin using mindfulness to soften the areas of my body that are tense or otherwise uncomfortable, and extend heart qualities of care and compassion to my experience. Sometimes this comes easily, but very often, self-love is hard to muster.

This is where qigong becomes an additional resource to mindfulness. Because the heart's job is so important, it has three helpers: the small intestine, pericardium (or heart protector) and the triple heater, which is like a thermostat in the body. This makes Fire a unique element, as it has four organs rather than two. Knowing this, I can draw on backup to help me extend care from my heart. I might start by softening and breathing into my small intestine, remembering that it is helping me distinguish between what is confusing and what is clear. I then send breath to my pericardium and help it be the shield that reinforces and protects my heart. I also breathe evenly and fully into my lower, middle and upper chest to help regulate my triple heater's temperatures. Understanding the roles that each Fire organ plays in supporting the heart provides insights into how our supreme sovereign meets its duties and continues to oversee our body, mind and spirit's well-being.

In qigong, there a few key forms that relate specifically to each of these organs. By understanding the specific role each organ has in the body, I have appreciated how the qigong forms related to these organs can optimally benefit my health and well-being.

The Small Intestine

The small intestine is the yang organ that pairs with our yin heart. The small intestine receives partially digested food from the stomach (food is also considered a form of qi) and breaks it down so that it can be absorbed into the bloodstream or released as waste. It is located in the abdomen, near the stomach.

In Chinese medicine and qigong, the small intestine also controls the way in which we absorb food and information. If we imagine that our heart is like the CEO of our body, the small intestine is that CEO's essential personal assistant: it filters through the junk mail, screens out unwelcome solicitations and separates the essential from the non-essential before passing it on to the boss.

When in balance, the small intestine does its job well. With food, it takes nutrients and sends them to the spleen, which then transports the nutrients throughout the body. Waste is sent down to the large intestine, where it is eventually eliminated through our urine and stools. Similarly, with thoughts and emotions, the small intestine sends the helpful thoughts to the heart, enabling it to make clear, measured decisions. The small intestine sends unhelpful, impure thoughts out through the large intestine, which relates to letting go.

When out of balance – for example, if there is too much happening and the job of sifting through material is overwhelming – then the small intestine becomes inefficient and sluggish. This can result in abdominal pain or problems such as IBS or constipation. Mentally and emotionally, we can also feel overwhelmed, leading to a confused heart that has a hard time making good judgements. With a healthy small intestine, we trust our gut. We also feel aligned with our thoughts and beliefs, and increase our capacity to see through complex, messy situations before they become sticky or intractable. Unburdened by indecision, the heart can radiate its capacity for compassion, insight and love.

The Pericardium, or Heart Protector

If the small intestine is like the secretary to the CEO, the pericardium is like a bodyguard to a president. While Western medicine does not define the pericardium as an organ, in Chinese medicine it is a principal yin organ – one that we cannot live without. It is the shield that protects the heart from the blows that strike it. Because the heart is so important in Chinese medicine, it cannot afford to receive direct attacks. Situations such as heartbreak, sudden death of a loved one or violence from wars or attacks are too much for the heart. It is, therefore, the role and duty of the heart protector to take the first blow.

Physically, the pericardium is a sheath around the heart. It holds the heart in place and protects the heart against infection. It also contains pericardial, or serous fluid, which prevents friction in the heartbeat. There is also a space between the pericardium and the heart, called the pericardial cavity, which absorbs shock and protects from sudden jerks to the heart.

Emotionally, the heart protector keeps the heart from feeling overwhelmed by all that happens around us. When in balance, the heart protector deflects tension and too much stimulation. When out of balance, however, it begins to absorb these experiences. This can lead to nervousness, anxiety or fear. If out of balance, it can also be too guarded – like an overly protective dog who barks at everyone passing his owner. A functioning heart protector is like a good bouncer at a nightclub: he keeps those out who might be offensive, drunk or might otherwise cause trouble, and lets in those there to have a good time. When the club is too full, he also prevents more from coming in until some inside have left. This ensures that the club is lively, fun and spacious enough for everyone to have a good time.

The Triple Heater (*Sanjio*)

Like the pericardium, the triple heater is not an organ that has an equivalent in Western medicine, and therefore is far harder to describe. It is a yang organ that is paired with the pericardium. It is often described as a thermostat that regulates moisture and temperature in three main areas of the torso: the abdomen, solar plexus and chest. The upper heater regulates the heat around the chest, throat, head and brain. The middle heater controls temperatures in our digestive organs, such as the spleen, stomach and gall bladder. The lower heater includes the liver, intestines, kidneys, bladder and reproductive organs.

If you have ever had acupuncture, you may have had your triple heater heat-tested. Often, a practitioner will place their hands on these three areas of the body and feel the temperatures. If one area is too cold or too hot, it can indicate a triple heater imbalance. My favourite example is the idea of a three-storey building. Ideally, the temperatures would stay consistent throughout the building, otherwise you might avoid one floor if it is too cold or burn up if you are stuck on the hottest level.

As a system that maintains balanced flow of moisture and heat between the upper, middle and lower torso, the triple heater also functions as a connector that lubricates and smooths out the interaction between different organ systems. This ability to create healthy links between parts of the body extends into the way in which we can also see our triple heater as the organ that supports appropriate behaviour in our relationships. A healthy triple heater ensures that we are not overly friendly or nosy, nor are we too aloof and stand-offish. A balanced triple heater fosters warmth in the way we communicate and create social connections. It helps us act appropriately in any given situation. For example, when we greet people such as our mailman, we say a pleasant 'Hello' and 'How are you?' instead of giving him the cold shoulder or showering him with questions about his family, friends, pets and past girlfriends. When we have a balanced triple heater, our organs are integrated as part of a whole. We also feel comfortable in social situations and at ease in our skin. We can also feel warmed by the balance of energy flowing through our body.

THE MERIDIANS

SMALL INTESTINE

The peak hours of activity for the small intestine are 1.00–3.00 p.m., a time best spent relaxing and allowing the filters to run smoothly.

The small intestine meridian starts near where the heart meridian ends – on the little finger. It begins on the outer edge of the nail, moves down the top of the hand and wrist, and then continues along the top of the outer arm until it reaches the shoulder. It then travels across to the front and base of the neck, moves up to the cheek, outer corner of the eye and ends in the ear.

PERICARDIUM

The peak hours of the pericardium are 7.00–9.00 p.m. According to the Chinese body clock, this would be a good time to spend in the company of our families, friends, pets or other loved ones.

The pericardium meridian begins in the centre of the chest. Internally, it moves through the diaphragm and emerges to beneath the surface of the skin just outside the nipple. It then flows to the armpit and down the inner arms to the elbow crease, forearm, wrist and palm. It ends at the outer edge of the middle fingernail.

TRIPLE HEATER

The triple heater is most active between 9.00 and 11.00 p.m. Before modern times, most of us would be preparing for sleep by 9.00 p.m. For many of us, today, going to bed at that time may seem outrageously early. For a Chinese doctor or qigong practitioner, however, it is ideal, as it enables the triple heater to begin an even distribution of qi through the torso.

The triple heater meridian starts at the outer corner of the ring finger and moves on the top of the hand, down to the top of the wrist. It then flows to the outer forearm, outer elbow and back of the arm to the shoulder. From there it moves internally to connect to the pericardium, resurfaces at the chest near the collarbone, ascends the side of the neck and ends on the back of the ear.

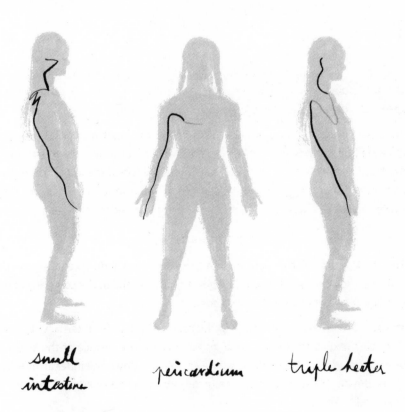

small
intestine

pericardium

triple heater

Practices for the Small Intestine, Pericardium and Triple Heater

Here are three qigong practices specifically for the three organs that support the heart. These can be done on their own, as part of other sequences (for example, the Eight Silk Brocades), or in the sequence I have outlined below. Each of these practices targets one of the Fire organs that our heart needs for health. The first form is active, whereas the second and third forms in this series are calmer and more meditative.

Two Hands Support the Heavens for the Triple Heater (*Shuang Shou Qing Tian Li San Jiao*)

This form is usually done as the third form of the Eight Brocades, but I like to practise it as the second. It is an excellent qigong form for balancing the triple heater. It also reduces stiffness in the shoulders, builds strength in the arm muscles, improves blood circulation and helps relax the body and mind.

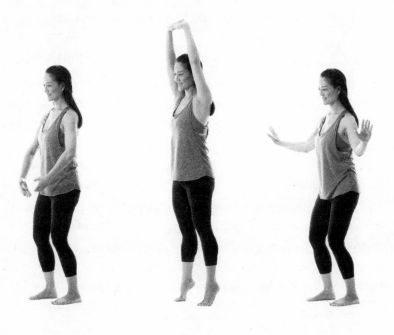

FORM INSTRUCTIONS

1.   Stand in *Wuji*, taking a few centring breaths that feel long, slow, even, fine and deep.

2.   Inhale and move the hands in front of the chest, palms facing the sky. Lift the hands slowly, interlacing the fingers at the level of the forehead, and then extend your two hands overhead, palms facing up. Straighten your knees slightly and if you want to, lift your heels for balance.

3.   Exhale and soften your knees, releasing the arms back down to the starting position.

4.   Repeat this movement for 7–9 rounds.

5.   Remember to keep the shoulders relaxed, and alternately bend and straighten your legs.

6.   Release the hands, and then draw them to the sides. Do one round of the Closing Form for Peaceful Qi (see page 61). Begin gathering intentions for integration, even warmth and feeling at ease in your skin in your two hands. Lift your hands overhead. Then turn the palms to face the earth. Begin to fill and nourish your body with your good intentions while simultaneously clearing and releasing any feelings of separateness or social unease that feel ready to be released. Fill and release with the hands until they return back to your sides.

7.   Stand back in *Wuji*. Observe how the body, mind and spirit feel.

Heart Protection Mudra and Meditation for the Pericardium

This is a standing meditation form with a hand position specifically for the pericardium. It involves a statically held position with the hands, which allows time for using intention and visualisation to direct the qi and support our heart protector in its job of shielding the heart.

FORM INSTRUCTIONS

1.   Stand in *Wuji*, taking a few centring breaths that feel long, slow, even, fine and deep. Maintain this breathing throughout the meditation.

2.   Bring the hands slowly and gradually up to the level of your heart, palms facing down. The hands should be about a foot (30 cm) away from your chest. Keep the shoulders down, elbows rounded, and wrists and hands soft and relaxed.

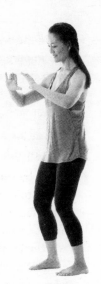

3. Turn the palms slightly out until they face away from the chest at a 45-degree angle. Keep the hands soft.

4. Begin your visualisation and intention practice: Inhale nourishment into your heart protector, such as the ability to absorb and deflect agitation, difficulty and distress. Exhale out what depletes it, such as things that shock the heart, cause anxiety and lead to fear.

5. Repeat for a few minutes. Begin with 10 rounds of breath, and gradually increase this to 15–30 breaths.

6. Finish by turning your palms to face the earth and lowering your hands slowly down to rest alongside your legs in *Wuji*. Observe how the heart and mind feel.

Separation of Pure and Impure Mudra and Meditation for the Small Intestine

This form is a meditation for the small intestine. The hands are placed around the gut to generate warmth and qi flow. It focuses on visualisations that can aid our heart's secretary to separate the pure from the impure.

FORM INSTRUCTIONS

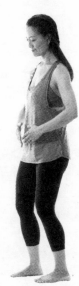

1. Stand in *Wuji*, taking a few centring breaths that feel long, slow, even, fine and deep. Maintain this breathing throughout the meditation.

2. From *Wuji*, lift your hands to the level of your gut, or the lower *dantian*. Turn your palms inwards to face your small intestine area. Point the index fingers and thumbs towards each other, leaving a small gap between them. Also let the hands rest a few centimetres/inches from your abdomen, where they can feel as though they are supporting your small intestine.

3. Imagine that the centres of your hands can transmit clean, pure qi into your small intestine.

4. Begin the breathing and visualisation practice of separating the pure from the impure. Inhale and imagine pure qi – whether it be clean, healthy food; balanced, clear emotions; or logical, lucid thoughts – into your small intestine. Exhale and let go of what is impure from your small intestine – perhaps indigestible food, difficult emotions, or confused thinking.

5. Repeat for a few minutes. Begin with 10 rounds of breath, and gradually increase this to 15–30 breaths.

6. Finish by turning your palms to face the earth and lowering your hands slowly to rest alongside your legs in *Wuji*. Observe how the gut, heart and mind feel, then do one round of Closing Form for Peaceful Qi. Extend the hands to the side, gathering clean, pure energy. Lift the hands overhead, and then turn the palms to face the earth, middle fingers pointing towards each other. Slowly and gradually lower the hands down in front of the face, chest and belly, filling with this pure qi. Simultaneously clear what is impure. When you finish, place your hands stacked on the lower *dantian*. Notice how you feel.

CHAPTER 10

Joy and *Shen*:
The Emotion and Spirit of Fire

Qigong is a practice that enables us to shift and move our body's qi so that it flows and functions in less chaotic and more natural, balanced ways. With regular practice, our body, mind and spirit begin to align with a sense of wholeness – the yin/yang harmony of the tai chi axis. It is a state that is naturally cheerful and bright. This instrinsic joy and brightness is believed to arise when the divine spirit, or *shen*, awakens.

Shen is the spirit of Fire. It resides in the heart and is believed to rise in the summer months. In its purest form, *shen* is divine light, relating to inspiration, insight, awareness and compassion. In the West, 'spirit' is defined as a principle of conscious life, or something that animates and gives life to any organism. We can feel free-spirited when we feel creative and unburdened, or we can feel spiritless when we are tired or sad. It is also understood to be the part of us that is non-physical, and the seat of emotions or character, or the soul. The same is true in Chinese culture.

Visually, we can explore the relationship of *shen* and Fire when looking at the Chinese radical for heart, *xin*. On the bottom, it shows the shape of an empty bowl. Above it and on either side are three small lines. The empty bowl symbolises a space where spirit can be filled. The three small lines represent the sparks of divine spirit. In Daoist cosmology, these sparks animate us at the moment of conception. They also awaken our consciousness and self-awareness.[7]

When we do qigong practices that help balance our Fire element, we build our *shen*. This can brighten our eyes, which is a sign of healthy *shen*, and increase our enthusiasm for life. When disturbed, however, we feel agitated and uneasy, like we are uncomfortable in our skin. Our eyes may become dull or flicker inconsistently. We are also mentally and emotionally unstable, which may result in seeking excessive pleasure or living an adrenaline-packed life. This all leads to an overburdened heart that feels too full.

As divine spirit, *shen* is light and requires space for expansion and growth. By design, the heart naturally creates space whenever its chambers alternately empty and fill. Spaciousness is often what the heart craves but lacks. We can easily overcrowd our heart with the burdens of life. In qigong, many of the practices are aimed at releasing what makes the heart feel too full and creating more space. When our hearts are spacious, we can feel inspired, authentic and connected to our true self. These are qualities that can help us through life and keep us open to the beauty and difficulty of love.

Love and joy

Love is a beautiful yet terrifying emotion. As Joan Crawford said, 'Love is a fire. But whether it is going to warm your hearth or burn down your house, you can never tell.' When we open up to love, we risk opening ourselves to becoming vulnerable and hurt. To love someone is one of the most courageous acts of faith. When we create the conditions for our Fire element to experience love in a balanced way, we are accepting that this balance grants us the ability to give and receive love, but also persevere through the difficulties and pain that love can bring. With a strong Fire element, we begin to love despite knowing that it will be lost. This is inevitable, and part of the cycle of life. With healthy Fire, however, we have a heart that can respond to this loss in ways that do not cripple us. We may fall out of love and feel hurt, but we do not stay heartbroken forever. Instead, we allow ourselves time to grieve, heal and – when the time is right – meet someone new.

Love most nourishes the heart. However, love is not the emotion associated with Fire – rather, it is joy. We generally consider joy to be a positive emotion. For the most part, it is. When we feel joy, we feel lighter, more connected with ourselves and others, and generally more optimistic about life. However, too much joy is a sign of overstimulation, which impedes the growth of *shen*. Imagine a child who is bouncing off the walls with joy to the point they cannot breathe or respond to requests to calm down. Usually, that child quickly goes from a fit of giggles to tears. This is the quality of Fire when unchecked: we burn beyond our capacity to abide calmly. On the flipside, not enough joy can also lead to feeling dispirited and broken, like a flame that is barely flickering. When we have a deficiency of Fire, we can feel cold, distant, isolated and afraid.

Joy in Chinese medicine and qigong is called *xi le*. The traditional characters for *xi le* reveal a nuanced understanding of what it means to be joyful.

$$喜樂$$

The character on the left, *xi*, has the image of a hand striking a drum, coupled with a mouth, from which we can sing joyous songs. *Xi* suggests festivities, excitement and elation, such as at occasions like weddings. In fact, when two *xi*s are paired, it is a symbol that means double happiness – a truly joyous occasion. *Le*, the character on the right, has the radicals for a drum. It is framed by bells and mounted on a stand. It represents orderly ceremonial music that is rhythmic and powerful, but never over-the-top.

Two translators of classical Chinese texts, Claude Larre and Elisabeth Rochat de la Vallée, describe *xi le* as the joining of elation and joy that creates a *joie de vivre*, 'born from the movements of breath whose ordered circulation gives an impulse that is unified in the heart and by the heart'.[8] Elation is exciting, whereas joy, as Larre and Rochat describe, has slowness, depth and tranquillity.[9] When we experience a balance of elation and joy, we feel a free and easy circulation created by Fire's warmth. Without healthy boundaries, however, Fire can get carried away quickly. Though much of our society advertises the need for thrill, thrill destabilises the tai chi axis and can be a quick path to exhaustion. When exhaustion hits, our Fire goes out, leaving spirit without a spark.

Finding balanced joy is like learning how to build a good campfire for cooking. You need a spark, some air and the right amount of kindling. Too much and the fire will overcook our food. Not enough, and the fire does not last.

Practices for *Shen* and Fire's Emotion of Joy

These qigong forms help nourish our heart's spirit and grow our capacity for a balanced Fire emotion of joy. These three forms can be done on their own, as a small sequence, or as part of longer sequences outlined in the Practice Guide at the end of this book (see page 231).

Lifting Ball (*Jian Qian Tuo Qiu*)

This form is part of the Tai Chi Qigong 18 Forms. It can be done as part of the full set of 18 Forms or done on its own. It is described as a form that can energise and lift the spirits, which supports our *shen*. The movements create a playfulness and sense of fulfilment and self-content that strengthens our overall well-being

When doing this form, imagine you are a child – happy, carefree and playing with your favourite ball. You might also like to see yourself as someone who is free and full of possibility. Invite your movements and breathing to remain steady and smooth throughout this form.

FORM INSTRUCTIONS

1. Stand in *Wuji*, taking a few centring breaths that feel long, slow, even, fine and deep.

2. Then inhale and step your feet slightly wider than the shoulders into a variation of Bow Stance (*Gongbu*). Bow Stance involves standing with the feet slightly wider than the shoulders with both feet turned slightly out and the knees bent.

3. Bring your two hands, palms facing up, to the level of the waist. Imagine each hand's palm holds an invisible ball that you can lift and lower without dropping.

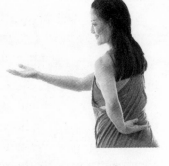

4. Inhale and cross your right hand in front of the chest and towards the left, lifting your imagined ball to shoulder height. Simultaneously bring the other hand behind you to the lower back, palm facing up, and raise the right heel.

5. Exhale and begin to release as you exchange the hands.

6. Inhale and begin to lift the left hand in front of the chest and towards the right, lifting the ball to shoulder height. The left heel can also lift. Make sure the shoulders stay relaxed and that the front hand doesn't lift too high.

7. Exhale, begin to change.

8. Repeat for 6–9 rounds. One round is lifting right and lowering, then lifting left and lowering.

9. To release, step the feet back into *Wuji*. Observe how your spirit feels.

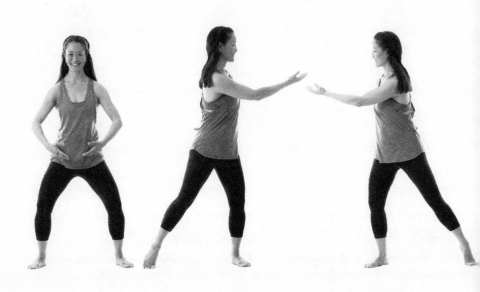

Flame in the Palm of the Hand
Mudra Meditation

As suggested by its name, this standing mudra meditation conjures the image of a flame in the palm of the hand. Holding this visualisation connects our mind and heart to the Fire element. We imagine that the hand is soft as it holds and radiates this flame. This can help to brighten our *shen*. We can also generate qualities of light, warmth and generosity, and invite them to emanate from our heart, which is like the sun of our body. This brightens the heart and can nourish our spirit, as well as foster our capacity for tenderness, care and love.

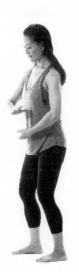 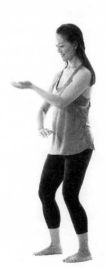 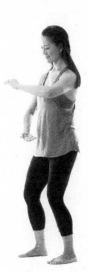

FORM INSTRUCTIONS

1. Stand in *Wuji*, taking a few centring breaths that feel long, slow, even, fine and deep. Throughout the practice, continue to breathe with these qualities.

2. Slowly and smoothly, start to place your right hand above the left, palms facing each other, at the level of the mid-belly. Imagine that your hands are holding something spherical. The top hand should be at the level of your solar plexus, and the bottom hand at the level of the lower *dantian*. Feel this shape for a moment, breathing.

3. Then, again moving slowly, bring the bottom, left hand forwards to the level of your chest and heart. Simultaneously lower the top, right hand towards the abdomen. The right palm faces the earth, the left palm faces the sky. The hands should align with your body's centre. There should also be a comfortable gap between your hands and your torso.

4. Visualise a flame in the palm of the left hand. Relax and soften the hand as thoroughly as you can. Invite the flame that rests in your palm to help warm, light and bring nourishment to your heart and *shen*.

5. Remain here for 5–10 breaths.

6. To change hands, turn the palms to face each other as though around an imaginary sphere.

7. Moving the hands slowly, bring the bottom, right hand forwards to the level of your chest and heart. Simultaneously lower the top, left hand towards the abdomen. The left palm faces the earth, the right palm faces the sky. The hands align with the centre and mid-line of your body.

8. Visualise a flame in the palm of your right hand. Relax and soften the hand as thoroughly as you can. Invite the flame that rests in it to awaken and enrich your heart and *shen*.

9. Remain here for 5–10 breaths.

10. Then draw both hands in once more and circle them around an imaginary sphere.

11. Slowly release the hands back down by your sides.

12. Stand in *Wuji* and observe the quality of your heart and its spirit.

Closing Form for Peaceful Qi
(*An Zhang Ping Qi*)

This clearing, gathering and sealing practice for Fire's emotion and spirit is similar to that for Wood (see page 61), but with an emphasis instead on the Fire element when in balance, and how this can support our ability to experience balanced joy. It is a classical qigong practice that uses intention and simple movements to affect the emotions and movement of qi through the body.

FORM INSTRUCTIONS

1. Start in *Wuji*, taking long, slow, even, fine and deep breaths.

2. Breathe naturally and with awareness in the *dantian*. Continue this *dantian* breathing throughout the following movements.

3. Turn the palms out and begin to move them slowly and deliberately to the sides and then overhead. As you do this, gather unnecessary feelings such as excess stimulation, anxiety, feeling carried away. These are ways that imbalanced joy and disturbances to our *shen* can manifest in our experience.

4. Once the hands are overhead, turn the palms to face the earth, middle fingers pointing towards each other, elbows bent.

5. Slowly and deliberately begin to lower the hands down in front of your face, neck, chest and belly. Use the intention to clear out the unnecessary feelings of overstimulation, anxiety and feeling carried away that are present.

6. The movement in Steps 3–5 then repeats, with a different intention: gather spaciousness, a *joie de vivre*, contentment and an uplifted spirit. Fill into the areas you have cleared.

7. The final movement is to gather all you have filled: spaciousness, contentment, an uplifted spirit. Seal this into your heart to help it radiate and shine brightly.

FINAL NOTE

Once you have finished all three movements, remain in *Wuji* for a few breaths, and absorb the way you feel. You can complete this by placing your palms on the lower *dantian* and noticing how your divine spirit and the emotion of joy feel.

PART 3

Earth Element

Nourishing the Mind

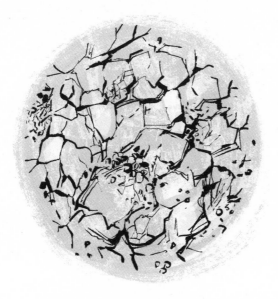

CHAPTER 11

Late Summer and the Earth Element: Abundant, Stable and Balancing All Life

After the pinnacle of summer's heat and before autumn's cooler weather arrives, there is a period when Mother Nature hangs in balance. This is known as the Earth season in Chinese medicine and qigong – a period that follows the heat of summer and precedes the coolness of autumn. In China and many agricultural societies in the northern hemisphere, this time is also when crops are harvested and people begin to feel abundance – a characteristic related to Earth in Chinese medicine and qigong. In the village of Sancha, late summer was when farmers reaped their bounty of chestnuts and walnuts, which fetched high prices in most produce markets. With their baskets full, there was always a sense of relief and reassurance: their yield ensured ample food and money to carry them through the year.

Earth in the Chinese Five Element theory

In the Five Element cycle, Earth is fed and nourished by Fire. Fire burns down to ash and builds earth. Earth also feeds and nourishes metal, and controls water by blocking or damming it when it overflows. Earth is also considered the yin to heaven's yang. This means that among the elements, its role carries special importance. In fact, among the Five Elements, in classical Chinese texts Earth is described as the most dominant of the elements.[1] This is because it supports and sustains all the other elements: it acts as the ground for plants to grow (Wood) as well as oceans, streams and rivers to flow (Water). Its fiery hot centre produces minerals from deep within its core that push upwards from the surface of the earth to form mountains (Metal). It receives and transforms the sun's constant outpouring of light and warmth (Fire) for life. In early diagrams of the Five Elements, Earth's supporting role meant that it occupied the centre.

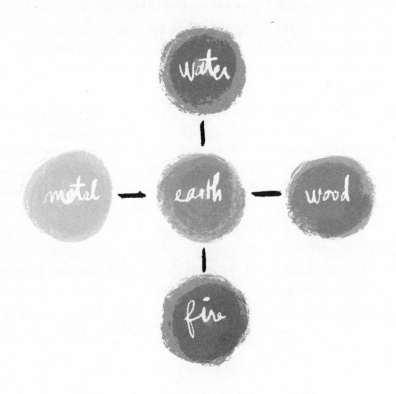

Earth's ability to balance and hold-centre

Earth energy in qigong primarily relates to the ability to be stable, balance and hold-centre. Like the planet Earth, which is always moving and transforming yet remains centred and steady in its rotation around the sun, we can work within our bodies and minds to resource the capacity for staying centred amidst the many opposing forces that may be at work in our everyday lives. The ability for qigong to help with this works in three primary ways:

1. **Movement**. From the moment we are born into the world and leave our mother's womb, our bodies navigate gravity. With qigong, we begin to explore this by feeling the connection between our feet on the earth and the crown of our head reaching towards the sky. We also work with the balance of rooting and rising, yielding and rebounding, or breathing in and breathing out. Through these interplays, we begin to imprint a more balanced use of our muscles, joints and bones. We also relieve sources of tension by soothing and smoothing out areas that tend to hold stress, such as our legs, back, neck and shoulders.

2. **Meeting our mental and emotional states**. When we take on too much, we can feel stuck, overwhelmed and ungrounded. In these situations, it can be easy to slip into a mindset of overanalysing and overthinking – both of which are signs of Earth out of balance. As we shall see in Chapter 14, much of our ability to nourish clear mental states rests on practices that nourish the spleen and stomach, which are Earth's associated organs. In Chinese Medicine and qigong, the spleen is said to house our thoughts and intentions, known as *yi* in Chinese. By nourishing our *yi*, we create an important resource that can help us focus and direct our mind.

3. **Meeting demands from everyday life**. Earth is the matrix that holds together all life. When we draw on this idea, we can find resources to help us accommodate the various demands in life from work, family and relationships. Finding this balance is difficult, yet by cultivating a more balanced Earth element through qigong, we can begin to align with Earth's supporting and stabilising energy. This can enable us to hold-centre amidst the many opposing forces at work, and find ease and harmony with the various demands we might juggle with the many constant changes and demands we face.

CHAPTER 12

The Power of *Yi* (Intention): Where Mind Goes, Qi Flows

In Chinese, there is a saying, *yi dao, qi dao*. This means 'when the *yi* arrives, the qi arrives'. This concept is central to understanding the importance and role of *yi* (intention) in qigong, which is understood most simply as our thoughts.

When we bring *yi* into qigong movements and meditation practices, we give the qi in our body a roadmap to follow. We can, for example, breathe in an intention to nourish the yin Earth organ of the spleen and breathe out an intention to expel waste and toxicity from it. With *yi*, we move and direct qi in order to nourish regions where we may experience excessive or deficient qi flow. Without *yi*, qi will still move and circulate, but far less effectively and with less potential to affect balance and healing. This is why *yi* is important in qigong.

In Chinese, the character for *yi* is formed using the radicals for the heart, the sun and the verb to establish or stand. When we integrate the concept of *yi* into any action, we can think of it as calling on our heart and the light of the sun to help our decisions. Understanding the role of *yi* is useful in understanding how we can feel qi.

Using the mind to direct qi

For most people new to qigong, the notion that we can direct the body's energy with our mind may be new and unfamiliar. This is because energy work rarely can be conceptually grasped or logically reasoned. Rather, learning to feel energy is embodied and highly experiential.

Here is a simple visualisation exercise to demonstrate how you might feel the way in which different intentions can change the experience of movement and qi flow.

1. Take your hands out to the side, turn your palms up, and simply lift them overhead. Notice the action of the hands moving up. Then turn your palms to face the earth, and simply release them back down, noticing again the quality of movement as they lower.

2. Next, take your hands out to the side again. Turn your palms up and imagine that a butterfly lands in the palm of each hand. With the butterflies there, lift your hands overhead with the intention of keeping your rare and precious passengers on your hands. Notice the quality of the movement. Then turn your palms to face the earth and imagine the butterflies walk to the top of each hand. Release your hands back down, with the butterflies still there, remaining aware of how your body moves.

3. Finally, take your hands out to the side, turn your palms up and imagine that your hands are holding heavy watermelons that are rather difficult to lift. Notice any resistance you feel as the hands and arms lift overhead.

4. When you release the hands, turn your palms out and down, imagining a large beach ball beneath them. Imagine trying to submerge the beach ball underwater. Notice how the arms and hands move, and whether you can feel any resistance.

Chances are, if you did this exercise, you will have noticed that with a butterfly in the palm of each hand, the movement slowed down and became steadier, more graceful and possibly more receptive. You may have observed with the image of something heavy like a watermelon in each hand that the movement quality changed. This is one way how our *yi* (thoughts/intention) can affect how we experience qi (energy). In using the intention to ensure the butterflies are not disturbed or the intention that the ball is submerged beneath the water, we can create a specific quality to any movement.

We use *yi* in qigong through visualisations. Using visualisations creates a depth and richness beyond the movement itself. Knowing the importance of visualisations can also support ease of movement, particularly through transitions.

Yi is also what I believe fundamentally sets qigong apart from other forms of movement-based meditation and healing practices such as yoga. For example, with yoga, we may be instructed to lengthen our spine, externally rotate the leg or firmly root through the feet. Postures such as Downward Facing Dog are named after the way dogs leisurely stretch after a nap. However, only a few new students I have seen trying the pose actually look like they are leisurely enjoying the stretch! Applying the concept of *yi* to the posture, however, could be interesting: if, while doing Downward Dog, we used visualisations such as rooting our hands into soft earth to enable our tailbone and sitting bones to lengthen towards the sun, like a diagonally blooming flower, then perhaps we would be practising yoga with *yi*. The pose, however, may require a new name, such as Diagonally Blooming Flower Posture! Only a few yoga teachers I know employ intentional movements or visualisations with the mind and intention to direct qi flow. Yet from a qigong perspective, making movement more healing might yield more positive results for the body.

With qigong, we have an ancient system for health that encourages us to use our mind to direct qi as we move, breathe and practise. Through this, we can also begin to explore the ways bringing *yi* into our movements can support our health and work to focus, steady and nourish the mind.

Practices for Helping *Yi* (Intention) Direct the Qi

These qigong Earth element practices use clear, strong *yi*. The first is a meditation that I often do standing, but you can also choose to do it lying down. Sitting is not recommended as it can be harder to feel into certain areas of the abdomen involved in this visualisation. The visualisation component of the practice helps quiet the mind and flow qi through the body. If you choose to do the meditations standing, you can follow with the second practice, which is a Monkey form. Monkey qigong forms draw on an external quickness paired with an internal stillness cultivated from the visualisation/meditation practice. You can do both of these forms on their own or as a set. However, if you choose to do the meditation lying down, simply rest after you complete it, and save the Monkey form for another time.

Meditation on Visualising Qi Move Through the Body – Standing or Lying

This meditation is quite powerful. The first time I began regularly practising this was after my second miscarriage. Doing this meditation not only helped me recover more quickly from the physical pain and hormonal imbalances that come with miscarriage, but it also quieted my mind from the onslaught of compulsive 'what if' stories that kept me searching for answers around my loss.

This version is based on a practice called Qi to the Four Limbs, described in Kenneth Cohen's book, *The Way of Qigong.*[2] I have modified his version and included intentional work to direct qi flow through the body. This practice involves bringing attention to three specific points in acupuncture. These are: 1) Bubbling Spring (*Yong Chuan*), located on the centre of the ball of the foot; 2) Meeting of Yin (*Hui Yin*) at the base of the pelvic floor; and 3) Origin Pass (*Guan Yuan*), located approximately 8 cm (3 inches) beneath the navel.

Bubbling Spring is known as a spirit point in acupuncture and qigong, where qi can move into the body as well as back out. It allows us to receive water at its source, and also connects us to our yin energy that arises from earth. Meeting of Yin is a strong point. It is where three of the most powerful meridian channels of the body converge and surface. These are the yin, yang and penetrating meridians (*Ren Mai, Du Mai* and *Chong Mai*). It can help balance many conditions, and also calm the mind. Among other functions, Origin Pass warms and tones the spleen, which is Earth's yin organ.

guan yuan

hui yin

yong chuan

VISUALISATION #1: BUBBLING SPRING AND MEETING OF YIN

1. While standing in *Wuji* or lying down, draw attention to your breathing. Take long, slow, even, fine and deep breaths.

2. Bring attention to the Bubbling Spring point on the centre of the ball of each foot. Inhale and bring healthy, vibrant, nourishing qi in through this point. Travel it up both of your legs to Meeting of Yin, the point at the base of your pelvic floor.

3. Exhale toxic, stagnant or diseased qi from Meeting of Yin back down through both of your legs and out from Bubbling Spring.

4. Continue, repeating this movement of qi up and down the legs from Bubbling Spring to Meeting of Yin. Repeat for 10–15 rounds of breath, or for 3–7 minutes.

VISUALISATION #2: BUBBLING SPRING, MEETING OF YIN AND ORIGIN PASS

1. While standing in *Wuji* or lying down, draw attention to your breathing. Take long, slow, even, fine and deep breaths.

2. Bring attention to the Bubbling Spring point on the centre of the ball of each foot. Inhale and bring healthy, vibrant, nourishing qi in through this point. Travel it up both of your legs to the Meeting of Yin, the point at the base of your pelvic floor, and then continue to travel this up to the Origin Pass, about 8 cm (3 inches) beneath your navel.

3. Exhale toxic, stagnant or diseased qi from Origin Pass back down first to the Meeting of Yin, before continuing through both of your legs and out from Bubbling Spring.

4. Continue, repeating this movement of qi up and down the legs from Bubbling Spring to the Meeting of Yin and Origin Pass. Repeat for 10–15 rounds of breath, or for 3–7 minutes.

Monkey Takes Earth Qi

This is one of many Monkey forms associated with the Five Animal Frolics. Most are complex and best learned from a teacher. However, I have chosen to include a form that is easy to learn, accessible and fun.

In China, monkeys represent clever, tricky animals that are nimble and quick. Their intelligence makes them fast learners and eager students. Their quick wits, however, have made them symbolic of our busy, distracted mind: just like monkeys who love to swing from branch to branch, our mind will jump from one thought to another and never enjoy the peace of being still. To train the monkey mind, qigong suggests that we cultivate a flexible, curious mind and heart that can be steadied and stilled through intention (*yi*) and will (*zhi*). As the sixteenth-century book by Wu Zhengen (Wu Ch'eng-en), *Monkey: The Journey to the West* describes, the most valuable teaching the monkey received from his Daoist master was this: 'Nothing in this world is difficult…it is only your thoughts that make it seem so.'[3]

When I practise Monkey, I always think of it as a cheeky little form. Compared to the other animals, it is playful and rather silly. Nevertheless, it yields good results for the body and mind. The form improves balance and builds strength in the feet and legs. It also works with alternately tensing and relaxing the muscles of the shoulders, chest, belly and pelvic floor, which can compress the blood vessels near the neck and head. This squeezing, pump-like action can stimulate blood flow to the brain and help quiet our monkey-mind tendencies.

When practising this Monkey form, let your movements feel light and quick while your mind remains steady and still.

FORM INSTRUCTIONS

1. Start in *Wuji*, taking long, slow, even, fine and deep breaths. Then, step the feet together.

2. Bring the hands to the front of the hips, with the wrists flexed and fingers spread gently open in 'monkey paw', palms facing the earth. Imagine you are a monkey taking in precious Earth qi.

3. Inhale and bring the fingers together, lifting the hands to the level of the chest. As they lift, the wrists flex quickly, creating 'grasping monkey paws'. As the monkey taking in Earth qi, you have grasped it into your hands and sneakily bring it up towards your chest. Begin to lift the shoulders, contract the abdomen, tighten your chest, and close and lift the muscles around your anus.

4. Hold your breath here. Shift your weight forward towards the balls of your feet and begin to gradually lift your heels off the ground. Keep your head vertical to help you find balance. Simultaneously look over the left shoulder, checking to see if anyone has seen you steal the Earth qi.

5. While still holding your breath, turn your head back to centre. Once you have seen that no one to your left has seen you take Earth qi, release your 'grasping monkey paws' and let your palms face the earth.

6. Exhale while lowering the released palms down. Simultaneously lower the heels and relax your contracted shoulders, chest, belly and anus. You have gotten away with your monkey shenanigans and can relax.

7. Repeat Steps 2–6, but this time turn your head to look over the right shoulder. Complete 2–3 rounds, left and right, and then release.

8. Finish by standing back in *Wuji*. Notice how the mind, heart and thoughts feel after practising this Monkey form.

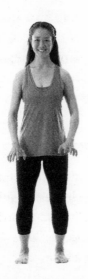
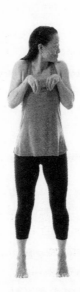
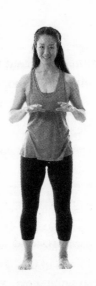

CHAPTER 13

Transitioning with Ease

The Earth element also enables us to explore and understand how it is we approach transitions, whether they be simple, such as moving from one qigong form to another, or more complex, such as when facing burdensome life changes. With qigong, we start with observing how we transition in the body. By learning to transition in more fluid, unbroken ways in qigong, we can, perhaps, also learn to transition with less resistance and more ease in daily life. This ability to meet change and not be jarred or have it radically offset our equanimity represents Earth in balance. When we are at home amidst changes large or small, we can feel a strong inner belonging and be steady wherever we are.

Earth governs smooth transitions

Unacknowledged by most of us in day-to-day life, the earth rotates on its axis each day, as well as orbits around the sun each year. Thankfully, these movements and transitions happen gradually and effortlessly; jerky starts and stops would be far less enjoyable. Because of the earth's dependable turns, we never feel this movement, even though it is happening every moment of our lives.

If only our transitions were likewise governed by similar qualities. For many, especially if situations we face are difficult, transitions mean disruption to what we know as comforting and familiar. Sometimes this is good, and some change can be welcome: getting a new haircut, for example, can feel like a fresh start. But often, even the best circumstances can be riddled with degrees of uncertainty. If we take a holiday, we may still feel anxious. Will I like my hotel? Will the food agree with me? Will I travel well with my friends or family? These worrying tendencies can be understood as an aspect of Earth element out of balance, which can be mentally and physically destabilising.

Unlike the earth, which balances opposing forces and is always smooth, steady and reliable as it turns around the sun, we often encounter transitions and meet them with a rough, wobbly and uncertain approach. Situations such as changing jobs, moving home, or falling in or out of love are difficult. Fortunately, in qigong and Chinese medicine, we can glean resources from the Earth element's transitional smoothness. This can support and help us meet transitions with steadiness and stability.

EARTH TRANSITION EXERCISE

This is a simple exercise of awareness of how you transition in your body:

From sitting down on a sofa, chair or cushion, simply stand up. Walk to the bathroom or kitchen. Then come back and sit down.

In these simple, everyday movements, were your movements sudden or gradual, choppy or serene? In qigong, all transitions orientate towards gradual, even movements – similar to the way the earth turns smoothly on its axis and revolves around the sun.

Earth Element Practices for Governing Smooth Transitions

These four practices support the Earth element's potential to help us govern smooth transitions. They work well together as a series but can also be done separately or as part of their original order in the Five Element Forms, Eight Silk Brocades or 18 Forms routines. As a short routine, I feel as though they offer a solid way to nourish our ability to feel smooth transitions.

Five Element Earth Practice

The Earth element practice from this series focuses on rotation, as well as movements that connect us to the balance of Earth's yin and Heaven's yang. In practising the form, each of our hands will move towards heaven as well as touch the earth. When you practise the turns, cultivate an ease and steadiness in your movements – just as the Earth element governs ease and smooth transitions.

FORM INSTRUCTIONS

1. Start in *Wuji*, taking long, slow, even, fine and deep breaths. Then step the feet together.

2. Inhale and step out hip-distance wide with your left foot. Simultaneously lift both hands to the left and then behind you, palms facing the sky.

3. Exhale and turn to the right. As you turn, let the left palm turn towards the sky, as if it is holding a platter. The bottom (right) palm faces the earth. Both elbows stay bent.

4. Inhale, look over the back (right) elbow.

5. Exhale the top left hand down to brush the earth.

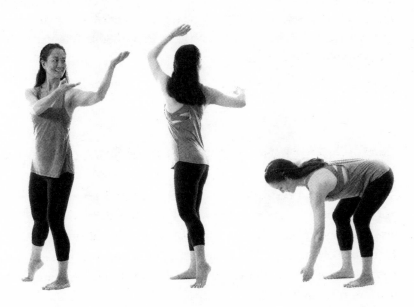

6. Inhale both arms out to the sides.

7. Exhale and step the left foot back in, next to the right, arms relaxing down.

8. Repeat Steps 2–7 on the second side, stepping out with the right foot hip-distance wide, hands extending to the right. Continue for 5–9 rounds, where one complete round is stepping the left and right feet out and back in.

9. Step the feet shoulder-distance apart one more time, into *Wuji* for the Closing Form for Peaceful Qi (see page 61). Inhale and turn the palms out to gather the qualities of Earth in balance: even, centred, able to transition smoothly. Begin to lift the hands to the side and overhead, imagining them filled with these qualities. Turn the palms down to face the earth and move the hands down gradually in front of your face, chest and belly. As you do this, use your hands to fill your body with the qualities of Earth in balance, at the same time clearing out tendencies to feel disorganised, jagged and choppy. Give these to the earth, like compost that can be transformed by the earth into something new.

10. To finish, place the hands on the lower *dantian*. Remain in *Wuji* for a few breaths, the feet soft on the earth, the head lightly up towards the heavens. Observe the qualities of the practice.

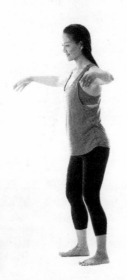
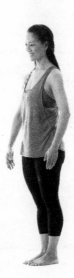

Looking Backwards to Eliminate Five Fatigues and Seven Illnesses (*Wu Lao Qi Shang Xiang Hou Qiao*)

This is the fourth form of the Eight Silk Brocades. It is also known as Wise Owl Turns Its Head to Eliminate Fatigue. It involves turning the head to free tension in the neck and shoulders. While owls have the ability to turn their head 180 or even 270 degrees, we are not quite going for that degree of rotation. Rather, we're rotating just enough to feel some space, but also to create hydration through the neck joints, without creating more tension or compression.

With regular practice, this form can begin to mitigate the effects of chronic tightness and tension in the neck and shoulders. It may also help us reduce the feeling of bearing the weight of the world on our shoulders. When we are overburdened and not able to meet life with stability, centredness and ease, it can be helpful to do what we can physically to create some space and reduce the load.

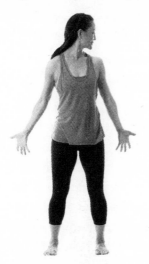 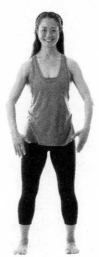

FORM INSTRUCTIONS

1. Start in *Wuji*, taking long, slow, even, fine and deep breaths.

2. Exhale and open your hands and arms to the side. Spread the fingers and palms wide open behind you, as the wings and feathers of a bird might fan open. Simultaneously turn your head to look over your left shoulder.

3. Inhale and begin to return your head to centre. The hands also turn back in towards the sides. Relax the fingers as they release down.

4. Exhale the palms open again, turning to look over the right shoulder.

5. Inhale back into centre, hands and fingers relaxed. This is one complete cycle.

6. Repeat Steps 2–5, keeping the movements and breathing steady and relaxed, and the head turning side to side as the hands and arms rotate. Complete 5–9 rounds.

7. After the last cycle, do the Closing Form for Peaceful Qi (see page 61). Turn your palms out and use your hands to gather conditions such as fatigue and stress-related illness. Lift your arms overhead. Then turn the palms down to face the earth, to clear the conditions, and move your hands down in front of your face, chest and belly. When we let go of tension and fatigue, we can perhaps do what this form is named after: eliminate the five fatigues and seven illnesses – or, at the very least, begin to mitigate the effects of tightness and tension in the head, neck and shoulders.

8. Finish by placing the hands on the lower *dantian*.

9. Remain in *Wuji* for a few breaths, the feet soft on the earth, the head lightly up towards the heavens. Observe the qualities of the practice.

Looking at the Moon
(*Zhuan Ti Wang Yue*)

This practice is the eighth form of the Tai Chi Qigong 18 Forms sequence. It is very good for helping to tone the spleen, an Earth organ, as well as the liver and gall bladder, Wood organs. It also increases qi flow through a spiralling shape in the spine, back and chest. Though the practice is quite active, the name of the form references the moon, which is soft and yin. During the Xia Dynasty (2070–1600 BCE), the first traditional dynasty according to Chinese history, shamans and sages were keen to understand the moon. They believed that if they could understand the moon's cycles of waxing and waning, they could also unlock the secret to immortality. These precursors of the Daoist sages sought to go to sacred places such as the Kunlun Mountains, or 'Mountains of the Moon', to attempt to unlock the moon's power and divinity.[4] Focus on smooth transitions and movements that come from a steady core and centre.

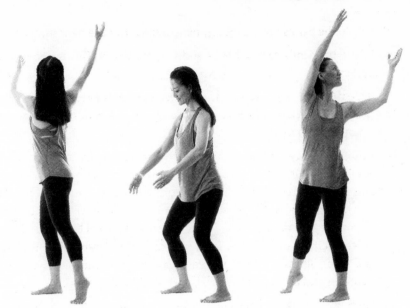

FORM INSTRUCTIONS

1. From *Wuji*, step the feet out slightly wider than the shoulders into a variation of Bow Stance. Turn the toes slightly out. Breathe long, slow, even, fine and deep breaths.

2. Inhale, lift both hands to the left and back towards an imaginary full moon in the sky. As you do this, allow the opposite, right heel to lift naturally. Keep the hands about a foot (30 cm) apart, as though shaped around the moon.

3. Exhale, use your hands to steadily bring the light of the full moon down in front of the body. Picture the moonlight reflecting on an imaginary surface of water. The hands should come level to the upper abdomen and the right heel should lower to the ground. Also keep the head and chest open and lifted.

4. Inhale, lift the hands to the right and back, towards the imaginary full moon in the sky. Again, as you do this, allow the opposite, left heel to lift naturally. Keep the hands about a foot (30 cm) apart, as though shaped around the moon.

5. Exhale, use your hands to steadily draw the light of the full moon down in front of the body. Again, picture the moonlight reflecting on an imaginary surface of water, and keep the hands level to the upper abdomen. The head and chest should stay open and lifted.

6. Repeat Steps 2–5 for 5–9 rounds.

7. To finish, lower the hands by the sides of your legs, and step back into *Wuji* for the next form.

Bouncing Ball
(*Tai Bu Pai Qiu*)

This is the penultimate form of the 18 Forms. It is more rhythmic than some of the other qigong forms described so far. It helps strengthen the feet and legs, improves balance and helps co-ordination. The movements can also establish balance between the left and right hemispheres of the brain, which govern logic and creativity respectively.

As you perform the form, the weight shifts alternately from right to left foot. While you practise, focus on keeping the movements steady and even, transitioning as effortlessly and weightlessly as you can from side to side.

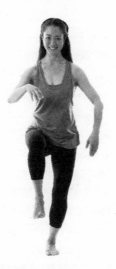 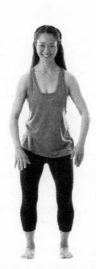

FORM INSTRUCTIONS

1. Start in *Wuji*, taking long, slow, even, fine and deep breaths.

2. Step the feet a little closer together and bend the knees.

3. Shift your weight to the left leg. Inhale your right palm up with it facing the earth. Simultaneously lift the right knee up, as if lifting your right knee up with your right hand, like a marionette drawing a puppet up by a string. Exhale the right foot and hand down.

4. Change legs. Inhale the left leg and hand up.

5. Exhale the left foot and hand down.

6. Repeat, and continue for 5–9 more rounds, stepping as if you were bouncing a ball.

7. To finish, step back into *Wuji*. Take a moment to observe your breathing and the hemispheres of your brain. Place your hands on the *dantian* and notice the effect of the practice.

CHAPTER 14

Digesting and Transforming: The Stomach and Spleen

For years, before practising qigong and receiving regular acupuncture treatments, I suffered from cold feet and hands. I also struggled with digestive disorders and was a bit more filled out than I am today. On good days, I tried to cheer myself up by thinking my pudgy body was like Yang Guifei, the notorious Tang Dynasty consort described as 'deliciously plump' by Chinese historian Charles Hucker.[5]

When diagnosing me, acupuncturists and herbalists described my conditions as Earth imbalances. The organs associated with Earth – the stomach and spleen – relate to our ability to receive nourishment, digest it and transform it. They saw my digestive problems as weak stomach qi, and my fleshiness and lack of circulation to my hands and feet as deficient spleen qi. On a doctor's recommendation, I began treatments and tried a new diet that supported my stomach and spleen. These helped to an extent, but it was only after learning about the Five Elements and starting regular practice of the Five Element qigong exercises that these conditions noticeably shifted for me.

From the Five Elements, I learned three things that quickly changed my Earth organ imbalance. One is the importance of regular exercise. Without movement, the stomach tends to feel stuck and stagnant, leaving little energy for the spleen to transport. The second is regularity and steady rhythm. Eating at the same times each day, going to sleep and getting up at consistent times, and working during regular hours enhance the stomach and spleen's function. The third is eating a large breakfast between the stomach's primary hours of 7.00–9.00 a.m. This powered me for the day, but also made the spleen hours that follow from 9.00–11.00 a.m. some of the most focused and concentrated hours of my day (the possible reason for this is explained below). Once I implemented these three lifestyle changes, my body's shape slimmed down and my digestion improved. I also began to feel warm hands and feet, which was a welcome relief.

The stomach and spleen also relate to our ability to receive mental and physical nourishment, digest it and transform it. When our stomach and spleen are in balance, we take in life's experiences and transform them into things that sustain rather than deplete or overwhelm us. We also integrate clear intentions (*yi*) that help us foster greater fulfilment and a sense of feeling at home in our experience, regardless of where we are or who we are with.

Let us take a closer look at the stomach and spleen, so that we can understand how qigong might benefit and support their optimal function in our body.

The Spleen

In Western medicine, the spleen's primary job is to filter and clean our blood by eliminating old, defective red blood cells. It also houses an abundance of white blood cells that filter out threatening bacteria that cause infection. In this way, the spleen plays an important role in our immune system.

In qigong and Chinese medicine, the spleen is a yin organ. Its role is to circulate qi by transforming what we ingest and transporting it as nutrient throughout the body via the blood. It may be helpful to think of the spleen as a grocery delivery van that picks up orders from one central storehouse and distributes them to different homes. When in balance, the distribution and circulation are healthy. When out of balance, we can sometimes feel cold hands or feet from a lack of efficient qi circulation in the blood. The spleen also oversees how we break down food and metabolise sugars.[6] This is why a spleen imbalance can result in carrying excess body weight.

The spleen is also believed to house our thoughts and govern how we concentrate and focus our mental energy. When our spleen is healthy, we tend to have undistracted and clear thoughts. When out of balance, we tend to brood and become overly pensive. When we overthink, it is like we are trying to absorb and digest too much information. This can lead us to become obsessive and worried, and cause our qi to become knotted and stuck. Because most human beings love to overthink and be seduced by stories, narratives and compulsive ideas, doing embodied, movement-based practices such as qigong or yoga can be extremely beneficial. The focus on how and where we move and feel sensations tends to bring us out of our heads and back into the present moment – an ideal antidote to worry.

The Stomach

The stomach is Earth's yang organ, which – surprisingly – we can live without. While having no stomach is not ideal, it is possible to take the stomach out and join the oesophagus directly to the small intestine and still digest some foods.[7]

Like the earth, our stomach is an organ that is always churning and turning in its efforts to process what we take in. Using the metaphor of the earth, if we feed the earth water, sunlight and healthy compost as nourishment, it produces abundant crops and foods that nourish us and fuel our growth. But if we put pesticides, toxins, plastics and other harmful substances into the earth, it eventually recoils and starts to show its fury as earthquakes, floods, fires and other harmful effects. The Earth can only take so much before it feels overwhelmed and needy. The same goes for the stomach.

The stomach's main job is to take the foods we eat and break them down, so that they can be absorbed and sent on as nourishment to the body. In Chinese medicine, this nourishment is qi. In both Western and Chinese medicinal views, what we attempt to digest directly affects the stomach's function. When we feed our stomach well, it breaks down what we take in as food, thoughts and emotions. This can be healthy food, clean water, positive thoughts and good company. If we feed our stomach poorly, it struggles to do what its job is in the body: churn and digest qi. No matter how strong our stomach muscles or potent our hydrochloric acid (our stomach has hydrochloric acid that kills or inhibits certain bacteria from food), it will be miserable if we overload it with poisonous foods, ideas or company.

SPLEEN AND STOMACH MERIDIANS

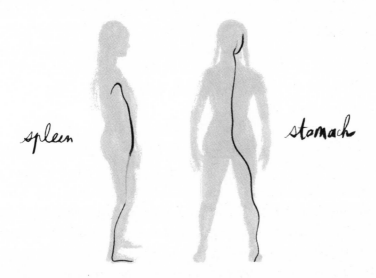

spleen

stomach

SPLEEN

The spleen's key hours are from 9.00 to 11.00 a.m. This is when food and qi from the stomach is transported and circulated most efficiently throughout our body. Because thoughts are believed to be housed in the spleen, it is also the best time of day for focused mental work.

The main, external spleen meridian starts on the outer tip of the big toenail. It then runs along the top of the foot and up the inner shin, thigh and groin. From there it travels up the abdomen and chest, to near the collarbone, before descending out towards the armpit.

STOMACH

The stomach's key hours are from 7.00 to 9.00 a.m. This is an ideal time of day to eat a hearty breakfast, as the stomach energy is strongest during these hours. By taking in a large meal during these hours, we also help ensure sufficient qi and nourishment throughout the day.

The stomach meridian starts beneath the eye, moves down the face, then splits off, one line from the jaw up the head, and the other down the neck and into the chest and down, up the neck to the head, and then back down across the chest, abdomen and outer leg and foot. It ends at the outer nail of the third toe.

Qigong Practices for the Stomach and Spleen

Here are three forms that help balance and support the optimal functioning of the spleen and stomach organs and meridians. Each is an active practice, which can improve circulation and movement for the spleen's transporting qualities. They also strengthen and tone the body's centre and core muscles on the abdomen and lower back, enabling the stomach to remain centred, strong and better able to digest what we consume.

These three forms are part of other routines such as the Eight Silk Brocades and Tai Chi Qigong 18 Forms. They can be done on their own, as part of these routines, or as the three-part sequence described here. As you do each exercise, let your movements remain fluid, strong and stable. While performing this exercise, keep the movements smooth.

Raise the Hands to Condition the Stomach and Spleen
(*Tiao Li Pi Wei Dan Ju Shou*)

This form is often done as the third of the Eight Silk Brocades. I usually prefer to place it second, as it feels centring and stabilising for my body and mind early in the series. It helps tone the arms, wrists and core of the body, as well as condition the stomach and spleen.

FORM INSTRUCTIONS

1. Start in *Wuji*, taking long, slow, even, fine and deep breaths.

2. Place your left hand next to your lower ribs, palm turned down. Your right palm is turned up and placed next to your ear.

3. Inhale. Then, as you exhale, press the two hands apart, bending the knees.

4. Inhale and change the hands, transitioning the arms smoothly so that the right palm faces the earth next to the ribs, and the left palm faces the sky and is placed next to your ear. Simultaneously also move the legs towards a straighter position.

5. Repeat, moving the hands in opposite directions. As you inhale, windmill the arms out smoothly. Exhale and press the hands apart, one towards the sky and one towards the earth.

6. Continue for 5–9 rounds, one round starting with the left hand pressing down and ending with the right hand pressing down. Alternate the knees bent and straight. Always finish with the right hand pressing down for balance.

7. When you finish, release the top, left hand.

8. From *Wuji*, perform the Closing Practice for Peaceful Qi (see page 61): turn both hands to the sides and begin to gather qualities of a healthy, nourished and balanced stomach and spleen. Lift these qualities overhead. Then, turning your palms to face the earth, begin to use your hands to fill into the form of your body the qualities of this balance: clear, focused thoughts and the ability to digest all that life brings. Simultaneously clear out tendencies to overthink and worry, as well as anything that feels hard to digest.

9. Finish in *Wuji*, observing how you feel.

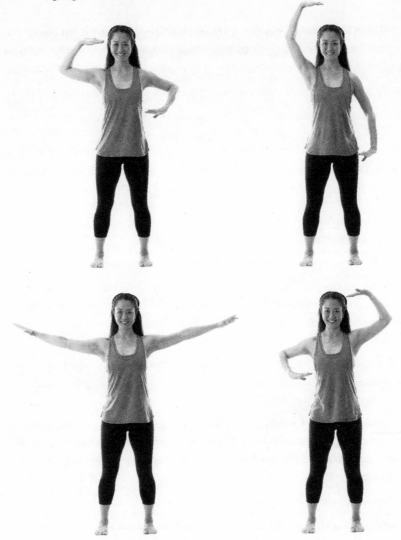

Rainbow Dance (*Hui Wu Cai Hong*)

This form is often included as the third in the series of the Tai Chi Qigong 18 Forms. In my personal practice and when I teach it, I prefer to include it as the fourth form, as the sequence flows more consistently this way. When I do the form, I like to use a slightly wider stance. The movement used in this form primarily conditions the stomach and strengthens digestion. It also reduces shoulder tension and is healthy for the spine.

Among the many benefits I appreciate about the 18 Forms is the imagery and ability to find relationship with elements of the natural world. In this form, for example, we are asked to imagine rainbows dancing in our hands. Rainbows appear when sunlight mixes with rain, and stretch from one end of the horizon line across the sky to the other. Normally, sunlight is white as it moves from the sky to the earth. When a sunbeam meets a raindrop and passes through it at certain angles, however, it creates a spectrum of coloured light that we humans can see and perhaps look at in amazement and wonder. When I see a rainbow, I am reminded that the Earth element's yin/yang function serves as the liaison between heaven and earth's tai chi axis.

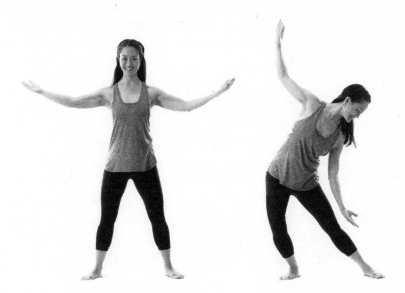

FORM INSTRUCTIONS

1. Start in *Wuji*, taking long, slow, even, fine and deep breaths.

2. Step the feet slightly wider than the shoulders, with the toes turned out. This is known as a variation of Bow Stance.

3. Inhale, open your hands to both sides, palms facing the sky, as if they each hold one end of the rainbow. Bend the knees and turn the toes slightly out.

4. Exhale, bend your right knee while keeping the left leg straight. Begin to tip down towards your straight left leg.

5. Inhale and rise up, imagining you can dance a rainbow between your hands.

6. Exhale and change sides, bending your left knee while keeping your right leg straight. Tip down towards your straight right leg.

7. Continue and repeat Steps 3–6, alternating side to side with your hands open and filled with rainbow light.

8. Release both arms down when you finish the routine, and stand with the head tilting towards the sky, feet on the earth.

9. Step the feet back into *Wuji* and notice how you feel.

Turning the Waist and Pushing the Palms (*Zhuan Yao Tui Zhang*)

This is the ninth form of the 18 Forms series. It benefits the spleen and stomach, improves digestion and strengthens the lower back. It can also help with backache and pain by creating greater support and integration through the muscles and joints around the lumbar spine.

> While you do the form, keep the knees softly bent and the shoulders and elbows relaxed. The palm pushes from an inner strength, the way you might use your whole body weight to push something heavy away, like a bookcase or heavy rock. Using inner strength will help develop and condition your core and consolidate around your centre for stable, strong Earth. This is an example of how to use *yi*, or intention, to affect the movement and energy in the form, or qi.

FORM INSTRUCTIONS

1. Start in *Wuji*, taking long, slow, even, fine and deep breaths.

2. Bring both hands, palms facing up towards the sky, to the level of your lower abdomen, or lower *dantian*.

3. Inhale, then exhale and begin to turn slightly to the left while you push the right palm out towards the left. Your bottom, left palm still faces the sky. Remember to keep the left hand at the level of the lower *dantian*.

4. Inhale, draw the right hand in, and then change the hands.

5. Exhale, turn towards the right while you push the left palm. Imagine you are pushing away something invisible yet heavy. This is using your *yi*, or intention, to direct qi. Remember to keep your right hand at the lower *dantian*, palm facing up.

6. Continue, and repeat Steps 3–5 for 5–9 rounds. Use inner strength to push.

7. To finish, bring both hands towards centre, palms facing the earth. Slowly release the hands down. Stand back in *Wuji* and notice how you feel.

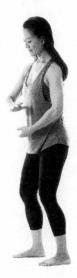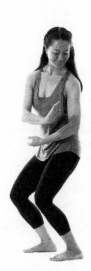

CHAPTER 15

Empathy and Trust: Earth's Emotion and Spirit

The emotion related to Earth is empathy. Empathy fosters connection; when we empathise with someone's misfortune or suffering, we establish a bond that helps us embrace qualities of the heart such as compassion, care and love. Like all emotions, however, empathy can be out of balance. When in balance, empathy creates trust, which is the virtue and spirit of Earth. With trust, we feel at ease. We relax into an acceptance and openness. We also feel safe and supported. When out of balance, we may care too much, be caught up in worry and feel like we are lacking important measures and means of control. Learning to balance Earth's emotions through qigong can give us back a trust in life.

In Chinese, the word for trust, *xin*, also means to put faith in a belief. For example, the word for religion is *xin yang*. *Yang* means upwards, meaning that the term *xin yang* can be translated as putting faith in something greater than ourselves. With Earth's trust, we begin to tap into a peace that comes with firm belief in someone or something. In qigong, this can be nature, harmony and feeling our tai chi axis align.

In Chinese medicine and qigong, trust is a cure for too much empathy. It emerges when our empathy is paired with genuine love and care. Yet, as we have seen with Fire's joy and Wood's anger, each emotion potentially can become imbalanced. Balanced empathy shows the right amount of nourishment and support for someone who may need it, like a mother who gives her child just the right amount of care and attention. Excessive empathy, however, is like a smothering mother who always worries and becomes overbearing, obsessive and unwelcome. How do we orientate towards a healthy emotion of sympathy and spirit of trust? By steadying our heart and mind, which is best supported by meditation.

The importance of meditation

When we are plagued by overthinking, worry and anxiety, we do not trust our intentions or actions. This causes our Earth energy to be negatively impacted. When we are free from these tendencies, our Earth qualities become steady and centred. Active qigong can shift our physical condition, which in turn affects our mental and emotional states.

In addition to physical movement, meditation is vital for Earth. The earliest Daoist sages practised *daoyin*, an ancient form of qigong, but also prioritised meditation. Zhuangzi (Chuang Tsu), for example, held that the physical practices were always considered inferior to more meditative practices such as 'sitting in oblivion' or 'the fasting of the mind'.[8]

Meditation is nourishment for the mind: it steadies the overthinking, overreaching and generally overactive tendencies of the mind; it focuses it. For many today, however, meditation is difficult, because our minds have rarely been trained to concentrate and focus for even longer than a minute – the monkey mind loves the stimulation of swinging wildly. With time, patience and commitment, however, meditation brings great benefit.

Practices for Nourishing Earth's Emotions and Spirit

These practices can help us create more balanced sympathy and clear intention in our body, mind and spirit. They can be done separately or as a series of four consecutive exercises. The only exercise that is part of another series of forms is the third, the Earth Element Mudra Form. This can be done with this series, or as part of the Five Element Mudras.

Spleen Meditation

This simple meditation can be done standing in *Wuji*, sitting on a chair, or lying down. It uses a visualisation to guide healthy sympathy into the spleen and discard tendencies for unhealthy sympathy.

MEDITATION INSTRUCTIONS

1. With your mind's eye, bring your attention and focus to your spleen: it is located on the right side of your torso, just under the right ribs. It is only about 13 cm (5 inches) long, and not very thick – perhaps 5 cm (2 inches) in diameter.

2. Inhale sincerity, understanding and supportive sympathy, filling these qualities into your spleen.

3. Exhale tendencies to smother, worry and over-sympathise, releasing them from your spleen.

4. Repeat this for 2–5 minutes, imagining your spleen's emotions grounded, centred and steady.

5. Finish by releasing the visualisation, and observe how you feel.

Shaking the Body

When the mind spins out and obsesses, we can get caught in a state of arousal and 'activation'. In nature, animals cope with aroused and activated states often by shaking. If you have ever watched a nature programme where a cheetah chases a gazelle, if the gazelle escapes, the first thing it does is shake its body. The cheetah, likely upset that it let its prey escape, also shakes. Humans used to do this after a hunt: we would dance, sing or chant. In today's modern world, we rarely shake, unless we are on a dance floor. Though it could be an urban qigong tale, I have heard that certain schools of qigong shake for up to seven hours at a time as a practice. For myself, however, a few minutes is usually sufficient.

You can do qigong shaking anywhere, any time of day. Generally, it's good to do before you begin other forms. I sometimes practise shaking after a stressful situation to help my nervous system recalibrate.

If you were sitting or lying down, please come to standing for this practice.

FORM INSTRUCTIONS

1. Start in *Wuji*, taking long, slow, even, fine and deep breaths. Maintain even breathing throughout the practice. Also keep the heels rooted down and the crown of the head lifted.

2. Begin a gentle shaking of the hands, using an easy, steady rhythm. Imagine your *dantian*, or abdominal centre, moving. The rhythm can be slower or faster, but it is important to keep the hands soft and moving consistently.

3. Continue, and shake from 30 seconds to 5 minutes. Keep the head level; resist letting it bob forwards and backwards.

4. To finish, release the hands down by your sides into *Wuji*. Observe any tingling sensations present in your hands; often, this is a sign that the qi is circulating and flowing well.

Earth Element Mudra Form
– Power of the Immeasurable Gods

The Earth mudra represents steadiness. The gesture helps nurture a sense of trust and security, like we know things will be OK. The steadying position of one hand at the navel and one hand at the heart centre aligns our centre at two important places of the lower and middle *dantians*. This can help foster a physical steadiness and remind us that we belong on this earth.

FORM INSTRUCTIONS

1. Start in *Wuji*, taking long, slow, even, fine and deep breaths.

2. Place the right hand a few inches in front of the chest, palm facing to the left side. Also place your left hand beneath it, a few inches in front of the lower abdomen, turned towards the sky.

3. Remain here and sense the steady presence of the top hand at the heart and your bottom hand at the abdomen. Remember to maintain even, long, steady breathing throughout the meditation.

4. After a few breaths, start to slowly exchange the position of your hands: the right hand moves in and then down and the left hand moves forwards and then up. The top left palm turns out to the side a few inches in front of the chest, the bottom right hand is a few centimetres/inches in front of the lower *dantian*, palm turned up to the sky.

5. Remain here for a few breaths, feeling an alignment and steadiness.

6. When you are finished, begin to bring both hands towards the centre. Bring both hands towards the solar plexus, palms facing the earth. Keep a few centimetres/inches between the fingers. Once the two hands meet at centre, let both hands descend softly back down towards the lower *dantian*, and then down to your sides.

7. Finish in *Wuji*, observing your heart's intention as it manifests in the worldly realms.

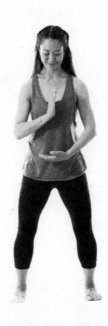

Closing Form for Peaceful Qi
(An Zhang Ping Qi)

Like the previous elemental closing forms (see pags 61 and 105), this clearing, gathering and sealing practice for Earth uses intention and simple movements to affect the emotions and movement of qi through the body.

FORM INSTRUCTIONS

1. Start in *Wuji*, taking long, slow, even, fine and deep breaths.

2. Breathe naturally and with awareness in the *dantian*. Continue this *dantian* breathing throughout the following movements.

3. Turn the palms out and begin to move them slowly and deliberately to the sides and then overhead. As you do this, gather unnecessary feelings of worry, overthinking and obsessive tendencies, which can lead to imbalanced sympathy.

4. Once the hands are overhead, turn the palms to face the earth, middle fingers pointing towards each other, elbows bent.

5. Slowly and deliberately begin to lower the hands down in front of your face, neck, chest and abdomen. Use the intention to clear out the unnecessary feelings of worry, overthinking and obsessive tendencies.

6. Repeat the movement in Steps 3–5, with a different intention, this time gathering qualities of sincerity, understanding and support, which are qualities of sympathy when in balance. Fill these into the space you have cleared.

7. The final movement is to gather all you have filled: sincerity, understanding and support. Seal this into your roots to help you nourish balanced Earth in the form of your body.

FINAL NOTE

Once you have finished all three movements, remain in *Wuji* for a few breaths and absorb the way you feel. You can complete this by placing your palms on the lower *dantian* and noticing how you feel.

PART 4

Metal Element

Nourishing the Spirit

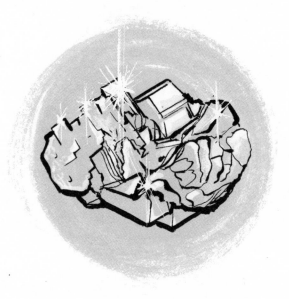

CHAPTER 16

Ascending Yin:
Autumn and the Metal Element

Autumn is a time for appreciation and nourishment of our spirits. From American and Canadian Thanksgiving, through the Autumn Harvest Festival in Britain and Ireland, to the Iranian Mehregan and the Chinese Autumn Moon Festival, autumn is a time when people and cultures appreciate a bountiful harvest with feasting, gratitude and generosity. It is also a time to take in nature's awe-inspiring display of leaves as they change from deep green to rich hues of amber, red, orange and pink.

Autumn is also the yin to spring's yang. If spring is nature's time for growth and expansion, autumn is its time to cut back and consolidate. It is the time of contraction, like a flower closing its petals. The leaves begin to fall off trees; the days grow shorter and cooler. This is representative of yin ascending: the earth slows down and prepares to rest. For some people, slowing down and resting do not come easily. Generally, myself included, people relate more easily to yang energies of expansiveness, lift and growth that happen in spring and summer than to the cold, quiet yin phases of autumn and winter. Viewed through the lens of the Chinese Five Elements, however, each part of the seasonal turn is essential to maintaining harmony in nature. Understanding these cycles is part of understanding the balance in nature and in ourselves.

Metal in the Chinese Five Element theory

In the creative cycle of the Chinese Five Elements, Metal is formed from the Earth's fiery core. The planet's core heat pushes stones and rocks up towards the earth's surface, shaping into plateaus, hills and mountains. Metal is also minerals, such as calcium, magnesium or iron, silver and gold. Precious gemstones mined from the earth, such as rubies, diamonds and sapphires, are some of Metal's more valued and rare manifestations. Earth therefore feeds Metal, nourishing it when deficient.

As a yin element and phase, Metal is solid, dense and structured – like a steel sword. This gives Metal qualities of power, strength and sharpness. Its sharpness gives it the ability to cut through Wood and curb unproductive or excess growth. It can also clarify the direction of growth. Metal controls Wood.

When in balance, Metal reflects determined, forceful and self-reliant qualities. People with good Metal tend to move past the frivolous and get straight to the point. They keep vagueness and confusion at bay, letting the doors to better judgement swing open. In balance, Metal's directness can be a virtue. Clear, motivated and straightforward thinkers are good decision-makers. When we have excessive Metal, however, we can feel too structured or rigid, causing Metal's strength to turn harsh, cutting and judgemental. When this happens, the Fire element can help soften Metal, allowing it to take new form. Fire controls Metal.

When we experience Metal deficiencies, we may feel unstructured and dull. Instead of logical and rational thought, we feel vague, unenthusiastic and afraid of being judged. This can turn into feeling unsure about ourselves and a general lack of self-confidence and determination. We will look at these tendencies in Chapter 18, which focuses on Metal's qualities of strength, dignity and courage.

Inspiration and letting go

Metal also relates to inspiration and letting go. We can understand inspiration sometimes more easily than we can understand and accept letting go. As with the beauty and preciousness of catching a falling leaf, we can find it hard to let go of what we consider precious or unique. We may also wax nostalgic for how much better things used to be. In today's accumulation-hungry culture, letting go may seem counterintuitive, or even an obstruction to our view of success. Being more productive, achieving new goals and buying newer, better technologies is the fuel of today's global economy. It also defines many of our social structures.

Letting go, however, is a natural part of the seasonal cycles and elemental phases. Without the leaves falling, there would be no nourishment for winter and growth in spring. In our everyday lives, letting go also enables us to begin appreciating all that we have. For example, when I go through my closet and donate clothing I no longer wear to charity, I'm left with the pieces that I like and value most. If we always hold on to everything, including things we no longer need, it becomes difficult to appreciate what we have in our lives. Similarly, if we let go of too much, we may also never appreciate what we have, or risk cutting ourselves off from people and things that can nourish, comfort and support us. Finding this balance can be challenging.

Qigong is an excellent practice that helps us work with the duality of inspiration and letting go happening all the time in our bodies. On a basic level, we work with this with each breath. The inhale draws in fresh, new air, the exhale removes toxicity and waste. When we combine this with movements that intentionally draw in nourishment and remove toxicity or waste, we can support our body's ability to absorb things that bring nourishment, and eliminate things that deplete us. When this process is at work in our bodies, it can begin to help us naturally appreciate what we have in our lives, and resist clinging to what is ready to go.

Slowing down, breathing and nurturing spirit

As the ascending yin cycle of the Five Elements, Metal also relates to our ability to slow down and see the true value and importance in life. When we are rushed, stressed, tense or trying to be productive every day, from morning until night, it can be hard to distinguish between what it is we treasure and what is of no value – be it the people in our lives, experiences or objects. Metal helps us to slow down. It assumes no one can sustain being as active as wood's growth in spring 100 per cent of the time.

For some, slowing down comes naturally. For myself, and many people I know, slowing down is not intuitive. Much of modern living is built around services, travel and communication becoming faster and more efficient. It can be easy to be swept up in a speedy race to express-mail ourselves to a finish line. While I still find myself sometimes going too fast, I try to live according to Ralph Waldo Emerson's wisdom: 'Adopt the pace of nature. Her secret is patience.'[1]

In qigong, movements are unrushed. Some may consider them slow, but usually the movements are not as fast as people may be used to. Because qigong uses fluid, intention-based movements, we naturally tend to slow down. This is, in part, because the mind and our thoughts can be quick, but usually the body needs more time to absorb the instructions given by our brain and central nervous system. Allowing the dialogue between mind and body to become balanced is a valuable outcome of regular qigong practice.

When we are less stressed and less hurried, we begin to breathe more deeply and feel more inspired. Breath is central to the Metal element. It relates to the lungs, which are the yin organ for Metal. The lungs draw in breath and qi, and, together with our large intestine and bladder (a Water organ), expel waste. Our breath is also one of the easiest ways to inspire and awaken our spirit. The word 'inspiration' is derived from the Latin *inspirare*, meaning 'to blow into', 'breathe upon', 'excite' or 'inflame'. In the Middle Ages, it also meant the 'immediate influence of God or a god', a meaning taken from the Book of Genesis: 'And the Lord God formed man of the dust on the ground, and breathed into his nostrils the breath of life; and man became a living soul.'[2]

In the following chapters, we will explore how we can understand qigong practices as supportive of our breathing, as well as other ways we can work to balance our Metal constitution, including cultivating balanced approaches to quality, courage and the emotion of grief.

CHAPTER 17

Cultivating Quality, Value and Preciousness

In mainland China, there is a cultural mindset known as *chabuduo*. It generally means 'close' or 'good enough'. It is a useful expression for when you make small mistakes, such as putting on two socks that both look black, but one is actually dark blue. 'Close enough' is OK when someone puts on mismatched socks, but when a builder tells you 'it's *chabuduo*' after installing a gas pipeline, there is cause for concern. In Chinese medicine and qigong, this runs counter to Metal's emphasis on healthy attention to detail. With good Metal, we intuitively respect and appreciate high-quality work, as well as the skill behind any action. In qigong, it means that we practise with integrity, without striving for perfection. We orientate our movements and intentions towards being even and smooth, rather than rough, random or coarse. I often think of quality movements in qigong like well-cut clothing: comfortable, fitting and elegant.

Finding value and preciousness in our body, mind and spirit

When we begin to cultivate good Metal through qigong, we can likewise begin to appreciate and respect investing in the preciousness and value of our physical bodies. Like polishing a diamond in the rough, we aim our practices at letting in light, and creating more space to reflect our inner radiance. Once we begin to feel this space and light, we may also naturally begin to safeguard this by monitoring our activities throughout the day more closely. We recognise that by making better choices about our exercise, diet and lifestyle, we begin to value, appreciate and respect our health and well-being more fully. Rather than short-change our body and accept a *chabuduo* stance about our body's life, healthy Metal helps us see the body as precious and deserving of good care.

Giving attention, care and respect to our body is not always easy. Since Ancient Greece, people in the West have tended to see the body as standing in the way of who we truly are, which is our soul.[3] Many messages in the media today are waging a war against our bodies. The body breaks down and needs to be sucked, tucked, trimmed, or exercised vigorously in order for it to be acceptable. In ancient India, the body was also not often respected. It was described in ancient texts as 'impure at birth…and impure also through death'.[4] One could only become clean by doing extreme fasting, breathing practices or other disciplines designed to radically purify the body so it can be liberated and free.[5]

Qigong sees the body differently. Rather than see our body as an inconvenient vessel that breaks down and generally causes trouble, qigong takes the view that our human form is precious. It also has the potential to thrive, even in old age. Sifu Matthew Cohen often says, 'Train for 10 years older than you are.' This means that at my age of 45, I train with the image of how I would like to feel when I am 55. I love this idea, because it respects the body as it ages. Rather than trying to reverse the inevitable ageing process and reject our present life, we honour our body and its natural ageing processes.

Metal Practices to Refine Qi Flow and Polish the Organs

I have chosen two qigong meditations for this section that invite the Metal element qualities of slowing down and refining qi through the meridians and organs. The first practice sharpens awareness and helps create a balance of yin and yang energies along the two main channels of the body, the *Ren Mai* and *Du Mai* (see pages 30–31). The second practice uses imagery of polishing imaginary gemstones in each of the five main organs of the body. This uses colours that are associated with each of the five organs and elements, and can bring significant benefit to the body's natural ability to defend itself from infection.

You can practise each meditation on its own, or use them together for a slightly longer session. You can choose to do these practices standing, sitting or lying down. If you stand, stand in *Wuji*. Choosing this option may be challenging if you are new to qigong, in which case, start with shorter sessions of 3–5 minutes, and gradually build up to longer periods of standing. If you sit, do so in a chair or on a cushion with your spine straight. If you choose to lie down, you may want to place a pillow or yoga bolster underneath your knees for comfort.

Microcosmic Orbit (*Xiao Zhou Tian*)

This practice is a classic qigong breathing visualisation. It originates from the Eight Extraordinary Meridians. These eight meridians relate to our deepest energetic levels, as they are believed to be the first to have formed in utero. They are also believed to carry our original essence, or *jing* (also known as *yuan qi*), from our parents and ancestors. The goal of Microcosmic Orbit is to create a continuous loop between two of the most important of the Eight Extraordinary Meridians, which are the *Ren Mai* and *Du Mai*, or primary Conception (yin) and Governing (yang) meridians of the body. When done regularly, this can help improve posture and strengthen the back. It is also believed that these two meridians are like main rivers of the body. By circulating qi more efficiently through them, energy will more easily reach the tributaries of the other meridians and organ systems.

There are numerous forms and methods of practising Microcosmic Orbit. I have chosen a simple yet highly effective approach that people of all levels of qigong experience may find beneficial.

As a caution, practising this breathing visualisation may cause light-headedness. If this happens, it is best to focus on the exhalation and grounding down through the base of the pelvic floor. It's also best to gradually build up the number of orbits and amount of time you practise this meditation.

VISUALISATION INSTRUCTIONS

1. Start either in *Wuji*, sitting upright or lying down, taking a few centring breaths that feel long, slow, even, fine and deep.

2. Place your hands stacked one over the other on the lower *dantian*. Begin to breathe into the space beneath your hands, imagining a coloured light filling and emptying from this space. The light can be golden-silver, like the yellow light of the sun combined with the pearl white of the moon, or a rose-quartz.

3. When you are ready to begin the orbit, exhale and descend the coloured light and your breath to the bottom of the pelvic floor. This is an acupuncture point known as the Meeting of Yin (*Hui Yin* – see Chapter 12, page 115, for a detailed description).

4. As you inhale, begin to let the coloured light move from the pelvic floor to the base of your spine, your tailbone. From there, inhale and begin to visualise the colour and breath rising up the entire length of the spine, including the lower, mid and upper spine, and continue moving it until reaching the top of your head. There is a point there known as the 100 Meeting Points (*Bai Hui*). This ascent moves along your primary yang meridian, or *Du Mai*.

5. Exhale the coloured light from the crown of your head or the 100 Meeting Points (*Bai Hui*) down the centre of the whole front body, which is your primary yin channel, or *Ren Mai*. Let the flow move along the front of your face, throat, chest and belly. Invite the movement to flow effortlessly downwards, like a stream, until it reaches your pelvic floor point of Meeting of Yin (*Hui Yin*). This completes one full orbit.

6. Repeat Steps 4–5 for 5–20 minutes. Let the qi naturally circulate along these channels in an ongoing and smooth orbit, in conjunction with your breathing. Over time, you can explore allowing the qi to continuously flow along these meridians with a natural breath that is not tied to intentional movement.

Organ Polishing Meditation

This practice is one of my favourite meditations and visualisations. It is based on a practice shared in Kenneth Cohen's book, *The Way of Qigong*, which works by sending colour and light to the organs. My own addition is the image of polishing the organs to reveal their innate radiance, light and health. From my experience, this practice has often helped me fend off infections and colds. In fact, if I do this practice when I begin to sense a cold coming on, through a tickle in my throat or general fatigue, 80–90 per cent of the time I keep sickness at bay.

The practice works with imagining the location of the yin organ for each element. In Chinese medicine and qigong, each element has a corresponding colour: Wood is green, Fire is red, Earth is yellow, Metal is white and Water is dark blue/black. For this practice, I have attributed gemstones that represent each of these colours, which supports the nourishment of our Metal element in particular, but will nevertheless benefit each organ and the whole body equally.

Element	Organ and location	Gemstone colour
Wood	Liver *(under the lower right ribs)*	Emerald green
Fire	Heart *(centre-left of the upper chest)*	Ruby red
Earth	Spleen *(left side of the chest, beneath the ribs)*	Topaz yellow
Metal	Lungs *(front and back sides of the chest)*	Diamond white
Water	Kidneys *(lower back/mid-back junction, either side of the spine)*	Sapphire blue/black

By using intention and visualisations, we can begin to polish the organs as though they were precious gemstones that become brighter and more radiant with each breath. Here's how:

MEDITATION INSTRUCTIONS

1. Start in *Wuji*, sitting upright or lying down, taking a few centring breaths that feel long, slow, even, fine and deep.

2. Bring your attention to the liver, underneath the right ribs. Inhale breath and vibrant qi to your liver and feel it radiating a deep emerald green light. Exhale out any dullness or tarnish, leaving the liver polished with a clearer and brighter emerald green. This can be toxicity, waste, imbalance or disease. You may also like to imagine that your exhale is like a cloth that wipes away dullness and restores shine. Repeat five rounds.

3. Now bring your attention to the heart, located inside the left upper chest. Inhale breath and vibrant qi to your heart organ, exposing a deep, rich ruby red colour. Exhale out anything that discolours or darkens the shine, leaving the heart polished with an effulgent and warm red ruby light. Repeat five rounds.

4. Next take your attention to your spleen, located beneath the heart and left ribs. Inhale and bring breath and vibrant qi to your spleen, seeing it become a brilliant yellow-orange topaz. Exhale out irregular qi, leaving the spleen polished, clean and smooth. Repeat five rounds.

5. Then bring your attention to your lungs. Inhale breath and vibrant qi to your lungs, revealing a brilliant diamond white light. Exhale out anything that diminishes the brilliance of the diamond white, leaving the lungs polished, illuminated and pure. Repeat five rounds.

6. Become aware of your kidneys, located on either side of your spine between the mid and lower back. Inhale breath and vibrant qi to your kidneys, which begin to glow with a deep blue-black sapphire light. Exhale out anything that diminishes this glow, leaving the kidneys glimmering with a polished midnight blue of sapphires. Repeat five rounds.

7. Finish by visualising all five organs as healthy, precious jewels that can glisten when held in your mind/heart, like the light of the sun.

CHAPTER 18

Metal's Dignity, Courage and Strength

When Metal is in balance, the associated characteristics of courage, strength and dignity become a rich resource for meeting life with poise and grace. In Chinese medicine and qigong, these characteristics are described as the archetypal father. Accessing this archetypal masculine energy, however, can be challenging. Many of us may feel we lack courage. Others of us may have been led to believe that strength should be resilience rather than virtue, aggression rather than compassion or benevolence. When we lose contact with compassionate, virtuous strength, we can become overbearing or even abusive of our power. On the flipside, we can also lose our dignity, self-respect and confidence.

Qigong and the Chinese Five Elements teach that each of us has access to an inherent self-esteem and boldness. These qualities drive our thirst for adventure, bravery and determination. They also help align us with what we hold to be authentic and honourable. For different reasons, however, these qualities may be dormant or restrained, which can be a sign of a Metal imbalance. To counter this, we can practise forms such as the White Tiger or the Flying Pigeon Spreads Its Wings, to help naturally awaken and release our inborn capacity for Metal's dignity, courage and strength.

Practices to Nourish Healthy Strength, Dignity and Courage

This is a four-part sequence that includes two White Tiger forms from the Five Animal Frolics, as well forms from the Tai Chi Qigong 18 Forms called Flying Pigeon Spreads Its Wings and Wild Goose Flying. I enjoy practising these together, as they harmonise the energy of a tiger's ferocious strength with a wild goose and pigeon's dignity, poise and self-esteem.

Both Tiger forms can be done on their own or as part of this sequence of four practices. I quite like pairing the Tiger forms with the Flying Pigeon and Wild Goose forms, as they balance movements of the arms and torso. Together, they feel structured and solid – qualities of balanced Metal.

White Tiger

In qigong, the animal associated with the Metal element is the white tiger. White tigers associate with many of the characteristics of Metal: they are rare, precious and also fierce and determined; they are brave, strong and courageous. The stripes of both the white and regular tiger symbolise ultimate harmony. Tigers are also heavy, grounded and quick; they can spring quickly to catch their prey.

With the White Tiger forms, we create strength and focus in the hands. We also condition the respiratory and circulatory systems, which support Metal's primary organ of the lungs, and increase tone through the arms and core of the body. While practising, it is advised to keep the eyes sharp and focused, like a tiger seeing its prey. Both forms can be performed with outer fierceness and inner softness.

WHITE TIGER FORM #1: WHITE TIGER BREATHING QI

1. Stand in *Wuji*, taking centring breaths that feel long, slow, even, fine and deep.

2. Shape your hands into Tiger Claw form, where both palms face the ground, fingers spread softly like the paws of a tiger. Imagine you can breathe in qualities of relaxed courage and confidence through your paws.

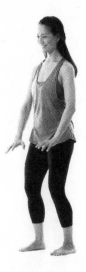
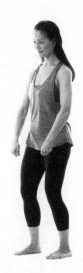
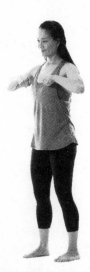

3. Inhale and begin to turn the hands out, making a soft fist by curling each finger in consecutively from the pinkie to the thumb, gathering healthy qi. You may also wish to gather resources for strength, bravery and dignity. Raise the fists slowly in front of the chest to the level of the shoulders.

4. Exhale and release the fists, extending the hands with the palms towards the sky. Imagine pushing the sky away with your hands, building strength in your arms. As you do this, let the hands transform into Tiger Claw hands, where the fingertips bend in and become like sharp claws. For Tiger Claw hands, keep the thumb, index and middle fingers particularly bent. Also focus on keeping a distance between the thumb and index finger.

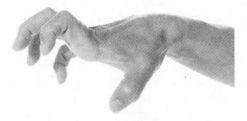

5. While still looking up at the hands, change the Tiger Claw hands back into soft fists by circling the hands inwards and curling in each finger consecutively, again from the pinkie to the thumb. Imagine you can gather qi with the fists from the sky that can give you courage.

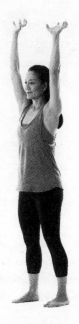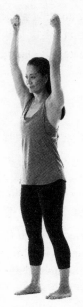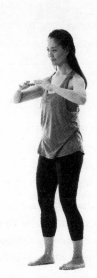

6. Exhale and begin to lower the fists towards the shoulders and chest. As the hands reach the level of your chest, gradually release the fists so that the palms face the earth. Lower the open palms slowly down from the chest to the abdomen, clearing toxic qi. You may also choose to clear out unnecessary harshness, rigidity, wilfulness or fear.

7. Return the hands by the sides of the legs, into *Wuji*.

8. Repeat Steps 2–6 between 5–9 rounds. Each time, let your eyes follow the movements of your hands, the body upright and strong.

9. To finish, stand in *Wuji* and observe how your body and mind feel.

WHITE TIGER FORM #2: WHITE TIGER CLIMBING TO THE
TOP OF THE MOUNTAIN

This form helps us with determination and focus, similar to that which we would need to climb a mountain. This movement helps us with mustering the strength to meet arduous work, difficult circumstances or fears. The tops of mountains are also where people across cultures and throughout the ages have gone to gain perspective and inspiration. Mountaintops also represent the Metal element's connection to spirit, as they soar high into the sky, often towering above the cloud line.

Do this form low to the ground, like a tiger climbing uphill. Use alternating arms and legs that might look like an exaggerated tiger walk. The arms also move like you might be freestyle swimming. The form benefits co-ordination and brings strength through the arms, legs and hands.

1. From *Wuji*, or after White Tiger Breathing Qi, take Tiger Claw hands.

2. Inhale, shift the weight onto your right leg, and step your left foot forward, toe lightly touching the ground. Simultaneously take your right arm and hand straight forward, in line with your chest, and your left arm straight back, in line with your waist.

3. Exhale, step forward, and lower the left foot down from the toe to the heel. Simultaneously rotate your back palm up towards the sky, and begin to gather qi in the hand. Roll this up and towards the front, as if swimming the arm forward and overhead in front crawl. At the same time, let the front arm lower down and begin to reach back.

4. Continue, alternating the arms with the opposite foot stepping forward. Move steadily, powerfully and gracefully, like a white tiger determined to climb to the top of a mountain. You can walk in a straight line or circle. Depending on the size of your practice space, take 5–20 steps. If you walk in a straight line, turn around when you reach one end and then walk back.

5. To finish, stand back in *Wuji*, and observe how your body and mind feel.

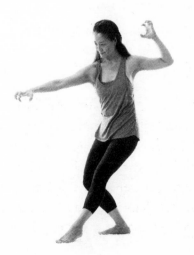
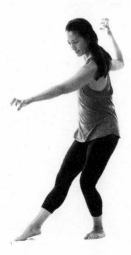

Flying Pigeon Spreads Its Wings
(*Fei Ge Zhan Chi*)

After doing the grounded, strong, clawed hand forms of White Tiger, this avian form feels like an appropriate balance of energy and intention. It conditions the heart and lungs, and helps to balance qi flow through these organs and corresponding meridians. It also strengthens the legs and helps open the chest. When we hold tension or become depressed or sad, we can unconsciously contract the upper back and chest. By gently opening and closing this area, we can begin to loosen it, which can help alleviate tension as well as mitigate tendencies towards depression and low self-esteem. This can encourage our intrinsic capacity to meet life's wide variety of experiences with less fear and more courage.

The name of this pose in Chinese suggests that the pigeon not only spreads its wings, but also exhibits them proudly (*zhan chi*). In this sense, we can connect to a feeling of dignity when doing this form. We can also feel degrees of self-respect and honour with our wide-open chest and wings. This is conventionally the thirteenth movement in the Tai Chi Qigong 18 Forms.

> While doing this form, keep your breathing steady and flowing, like the movements of a bird in flight. Also keep the hands soft, light and relaxed, as though made of feathers.

FORM INSTRUCTIONS

1. Stand in *Wuji*, taking centring breaths that feel long, slow, even, fine and deep.

2. Exhale and step your right foot forward.

3. Gently rock your weight forward, bend the right knee, and allow your back heel to lift. At the same time, move your outstretched arms forwards in front of your chest, like the wings of a pigeon closing. The hands, however, do not cross or touch, even though they move towards each other.

4. Inhale and gently rock your weight back, bending the back knee and lifting the front toes. Simultaneously open your arms to the sides and back, as if spreading your wings. This will open your chest, and is one complete round.

5. Continue, rocking forward. Repeat Steps 3–4 for 6–9 rounds.

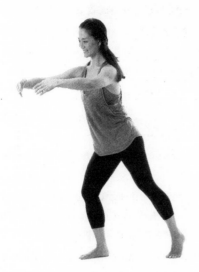
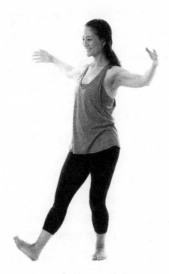

6. Change the feet, and begin again on the second side, with the left foot forward and right foot back. Do 6–9 rounds on the left.

7. To finish, step the front foot back in and stand in *Wuji*. Notice how the breath and body feel.

Wild Goose Flying (*Da Yan Fei Xiang*)

In China, wild geese (as distinct from domesticated geese) symbolise fidelity, as well as seasonal migration and change. Their long, northern spring migrations are taken to avoid the rising yang heat of summer; their equally long autumn southern migrations to avoid the cold and dark of winter's yin. In this way, geese are seen to be part of the manifestations of yin and yang energies. Their annual autumn migrations in particular have been the subject of Chinese poems and paintings from the Han Dynasty onwards (206 BCE–221 CE). When wild geese fly south, it indicates the arrival of autumn and its forces of yin rising, which is when the harvest should begin.[6] When we do this practice, we might imagine that when we open our wild goose wings, we do so with a natural sense of purpose and determination of a southern flight.

Traditionally, this form is the fifteenth of the 18 Tai Chi Qigong Forms. When I practise the 18 Forms, however, I tend to do it as the fourteenth form. The gentle opening and closing cools and begins to quiet our body and mind. It is believed that this form helps qi expand through the upper chest and lungs. It can also help relieve headaches and reduce the effects of mental stress and chronic nervous disorders.

FORM INSTRUCTIONS

1. Start in *Wuji*, taking long, slow, even, fine and deep breaths.

2. Then step the feet together, letting the inner edges of your toes and heels touch.

3. Inhale and lift the arms to the sides, palms turned slightly out, to shoulder height. The legs stay steady as the hands reach out. Allow the arms to lift less from your hands and more from a sense that the underarms expand.

4. Let the fingers extend and then point slightly towards the sky at about a 45-degree angle. This will gently stretch the fingers in the opposite direction of the Tiger Claw hand form.

5. Exhale, retract the elbows and wrists, and gradually release the hands down like soft, feathering wings to the sides of your body.

6. Repeat Steps 3–5 for 6–9 rounds.

7. To finish, stand in *Wuji*, observing how your body feels.

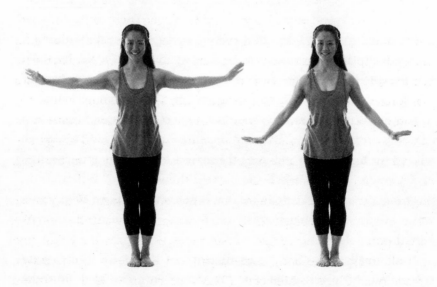

CHAPTER 19

Metal's Organs:
The Lungs and Large Intestine

For most of my life, I have had weak lungs. This was in part due to early childhood illnesses such as asthma, pneumonia and bronchitis. In fact, as a child, I was so fragile that my parents chose to move our family from upstate New York to the dry, hot desert of Tucson, Arizona, in the hope that the arid climate would improve my health. My asthma only worsened, though. Fortunately, when I was eight years old, I began a daily regime of Chinese herbs that abated the condition completely for a number of years. As an adult, however, my asthma came back, with a cruel vengeance.

Looking back, I can see that my health problems were closely tied to the Metal element, which in Chinese medicine and qigong relates to the lungs as well as the large intestine. When I was in the throes of my asthmatic recurrence, I did everything I shouldn't do for my poor lungs: I smoked, rarely exercised and ate foods that were hard to digest. As a result, my lungs and large intestine struggled with inefficiency for far longer than necessary. Constipation was also a constant worry, and I had dry skin and cracking joints – other signs of Metal imbalances. Once I started doing regular yoga, my digestion improved marginally, as did my asthma. Despite yoga's emphasis on breathing, surprisingly, my lungs remained fairly weak.

After I learned about Chinese medicine and qigong, I began to see that with the Metal phase there is an orientation towards dryness. We see autumn's dryness unfold in nature, as leaves become brittle and fall off trees. In the body, some drying out is healthy and necessary. Traditional Chinese Medicine (TCM) practitioner Gail Reichstein describes how Metal's dryness 'filters breath through the lungs and food mass through the bowels to isolate their essence and eliminate impurities'.[7] Too much, however, 'renders us as cracked and vulnerable as a droughty plain'.[8] Our skin can become parched and cracked, our joints creaky and juiceless. Conversely, an inability to dry out excess fluids can also result in too much mucus and phlegm.

In their efforts to try to regulate the moisture levels in my chest, my lungs took charge of my whole body. Like an efficient minister, they order all organs to try to comply with their wishes, particularly the large intestine and Metal's sense organ, the skin. In my case, my lungs were desperately trying to dry out the fluid inside of them, but they were too weak to do an effective job. Nevertheless, their effort to dry resulted in my whole body dehydrating to try to compensate.

Unfortunately, the type of dryness caused by Metal is not just remedied by drinking more water. To keep the effects of Metal's overly drying tendencies in check, there is little better than the slow, fluid movements of qigong and tai chi chuan, which nourish rather than overexert the body. Moreover, as much as I loved my yoga, my approach at the time was too vigorous and heating. With regular qigong practice, however, many of my symptoms of imbalanced Metal subsided. Though my joints still occasionally crack and my skin is still prone to dryness, my asthma has nearly disappeared and I am no longer plagued by constipation. While I am still cautious about asthma and know my lungs are susceptible to weakness, I now feel armed with tools and practices from qigong and Five Element wisdom to help me keep them healthier and more balanced.

The Lungs

The lungs are the yin organ of Metal. In classical Chinese texts on medicine, they are described as holding the 'office of minister and chancellor'.[9] This is because next to the heart, the lungs are the most important organ in the body. They are like the top advisor to the sovereign, helping the heart in regulating the body's qi. When they function well, they balance and disperse fluids in the body, preparing them to be eliminated by the large intestine as well as through actions like urinating or sweating. When weak, their ability to do this is impaired. This can lead to a build-up of phlegm and mucus. The lungs also receive a large supply of blood directly from the heart; no other organ receives this in as high a quantity as the lungs.[10]

In Western medicine, the pair of lungs are the primary organ for respiration. Their job is exchanging carbon dioxide for oxygen. To do this, they draw in oxygen from the air on the inhale, transfer it into the bloodstream, and then release carbon dioxide from the bloodstream back into the air on the exhale. This is why, when breathing, we should always give equal emphasis to the in breath but also to the out breath. Every time you exhale, you release up to 70 per cent of your body's toxicity.[11] This is also why, among other reasons, it is important to use long, slow, even, fine and deep breathing not only in qigong practice but also in daily life.

Though the lungs have a large capacity for breath, they are considered a delicate organ in Chinese medicine. They are like the leaves on a tree, easily damaged by dryness as well as excess fluid. The structure of the branches and bronchial tubes inside the lungs looks like an inverted tree. Acupuncturist and Western MD Daniel Keown describes the process trees use to carry nutrients from the sun and transport them through the tree and its roots as nearly identical to how the lungs function in our body. The difference, he notes, is that 'sunlight is to trees what spirit is to our lungs'.[12]

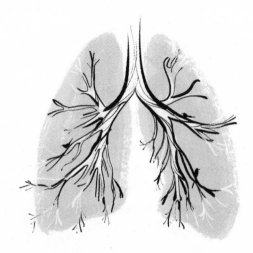

THE IMPORTANCE OF BREATHING:
SPIRIT, PURE QI AND THE LUNGS

In Chinese medicine and qigong, spirit requires the lungs' exacting refinement to extract the purest qualities from the air they breathe in and distribute this to the body. In qigong, this pure essence is refined qi. The lungs are believed to take in pure qi from heaven, and are therefore our closest connection to spirit. In this sense, the lungs nourish our spirit through the ordinary yet extraordinary act of breathing.

For humans, breath affects our mental and emotional states. Our mental and emotional states also affect our breath. When we are excited, we gasp; tired, we sigh. When we are nervous or scared, our breathing tends to quicken; relaxed and calm, our breath slows and deepens. Yet we can also change our breathing at will. If we recognise moments when we are anxious or tense and begin to take long, slow, deep breaths, we tend to calm down. All of these actions affect our spirit.

When our breathing function is impaired, we can feel fatigued or suffer from conditions such as respiratory disorders, asthma, dry skin and constipation. This may lead us to feel dispirited, moody, dull and uninspired. When our breathing patterns are healthy, we will feel energised and more inspired by life. In qigong, we can support this by ensuring we have sufficient pure qi to nourish our breath and, therefore, our spirit.

Large Intestine

Like the exhaling action of the lungs, the large intestine is responsible for transporting and eliminating waste as stools. In Chinese medicine and qigong, it is the yang organ paired with the yin lungs. As such, it continues the drying process started by the lungs, by converting digestive waste from fluids to solids that can be released. It also assists the lungs in balancing these fluids, and ensures the purity of qi in the body by removing that which is no longer needed by the body.

The large intestine is also known as the colon. It is the last part of the digestive tract in humans and other vertebrates. In Western medicine, the colon's primary job is similar to that in Chinese medicine: it extracts and absorbs water as well as salt from food waste, storing what is left as stools before they are released. The colon is located in the pelvic bowl beneath the waist, and has three sections: the ascending, transverse and descending aspects. The ascending colon is on the right side of the lower abdomen, the transverse across the top and descending on the left side. It is about 1.5 metres (5 feet) long and 5–8 cm (2–3 inches) thick. In qigong, there are some self-massage techniques that involve moving the hands in a clockwise direction around the abdomen, to help the large intestine's work of digestion and elimination.

THE LUNGS AND LARGE INTESTINE MERIDIANS

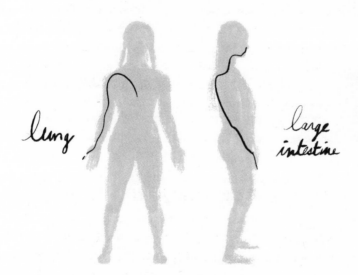

lung

large intestine

LUNGS

The lungs are most active during the early morning hours of 3.00–5.00 a.m. In many spiritual traditions such as Buddhism and yoga, these early morning hours are the best times to meditate or practise breathing exercises. In Chinese medicine and qigong, however, you would ideally still be asleep during the lung hours, to maximise rest.

The lung meridian runs from the chest to beneath the mid-collarbone, across to the shoulder and down the inner arm, where it continues along to the base of the thumb and outer thumbnail.

LARGE INTESTINE

The large intestine hours are 5.00–7.00 a.m. This is an ideal time of day to have a bowel movement and release the digested waste that is ready to move out of the body.

The large intestine meridian begins on the outer fingernail of the index finger. It then moves up the finger and top of the hand to the space between the thumb and index finger, up the wrist, forearm, outer elbow and outer upper arm. It then travels to the shoulder, side of the neck, cheek, lower gums and top lip, ending beside the nostril.

Practices to Nourish the Lungs and Large Intestine

This set of three qigong forms combines practices from the Five Elements qigong series, the Tai Chi Qigong 18 Forms and the Eight Silk Brocades. The forms can be done as part of these other sequences, on their own, or in this sequence of three postures for Metal. By putting these three forms together, we can target the organs for Metal more specifically, and help their optimal function.

Five Element Metal Practice

This is part of the Five Elements qigong forms. It works specifically with the organs of our lungs and large intestine. It invites us into a connection to the vital resource of our breath. In this way, we support our body's ability to breathe in what inspires and nourishes us, and let go of what depletes us and holds us back. We also open up to the potential of transformation, inspiration and purity. The practice strengthens the muscles around the lungs and mid-back, and gently conditions the arms and legs.

FORM INSTRUCTIONS

1. Start in *Wuji*, taking long, slow, even, fine and deep breaths.

2. Step the feet together, hands by your sides.

3. Inhale and step your left foot out to shoulder-distance wide. Simultaneously lift your hands forwards, palms facing the sky as if gathering qi. Continue on the in-breath to draw your hands in, bending the elbows back so that the hands come to the two sides of your lungs and chest.

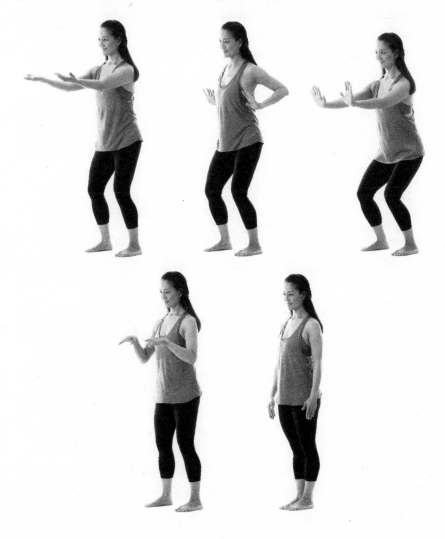

4. Exhale, bend the knees and press the palms forwards, from the sides of the ribs and lungs.

5. Inhale, lift from the crown of your head to straighten the legs. Simultaneously draw the arms and hands softly in towards your chest, keeping the hands relaxed and palms facing the earth.

6. Exhale and begin to release the hands down as though you could release toxicity. Also step the left foot back in, next to the right.

7. Repeat Steps 3–6 to the second side, stepping out with the right foot. When you complete this round, step the right foot back in. This is one full cycle.

8. Continue for 5–9 rounds. With each inhale, imagine drawing healthy, vibrant qi into your lungs, and with each exhale, letting go of toxic or stagnant qi. You can also work with drawing in inspiration as you inhale, and exhaling out what weighs you down.

9. Step the feet back out, into *Wuji*.

10. Perform one round of the Closing Form for Peaceful Qi (see page 61): Extend the palms to the sides and begin to gather healthy lung qi with your hands. Lift them overhead, and then begin to turn the palms towards the earth. Lower the hands gradually down in front of your face, throat, lungs and large intestine, filling with clean, healthy qi for your lungs. Imagine clearing out any residual toxicity or waste that may have been stirred up from the movement.

11. Finish by replacing the hands on the *dantian*. Breathe, noticing the effect of the Metal element form in the body.

Touch the Sea, Look at the Sky
(*Lao Hai Guan Tian*)

This form is traditionally the eleventh of the Tai Chi Qigong 18 Forms. It blends the large intestine's qualities of letting go towards an imaginary sea, with the lungs' capacity to fill and find connection to the sky – home to spirit and heaven. The form primarily benefits the lungs and large intestine meridians with the opening and closing movements of the arms, abdomen and chest, but it also supports the healthy functioning of the spleen, heart and kidneys, and can help strengthen the legs, waist and back.

The sequence also helps balance the body's yin and yang aspects. When we bend forwards and feel connected to the softness and depth of the sea, this is yin. When we lift upwards and extend towards the sky, this is yang. As such, it is a form that helps us harmonise yin and yang, and feel closer to the tai chi axis of balance.

> When performing the movements, imagine that you are standing at the top of a mountain, with the openness of the sky all around you, and then dive down to touch the sea. The imagery and movements of expansion and contraction make this one of my favourite forms.

FORM INSTRUCTIONS

1. From *Wuji* (picking up from Five Element Metal Practice), take a few long, slow, even, fine and deep breaths.

2. Then step your right foot forwards, about one foot (30 cm) away, into a variation of Bow Stance. You should be able to back-weight and bend your back left leg, without straining your knee. You should also be able to bend your front right knee and not have it go too far over the ankle.

3. Exhale and begin to cross your arms in front of your right shin.

4. Keeping your arms still crossing, inhale and stand up, shifting your weight to bend the back knee. Once your crossed arms reach overhead, open them to the sides, looking at the sky.

5. Repeat Steps 3–4. Exhale and bend your front knee. Cross the hands, touching the cool waters of the yin sea. Inhale, coming up, bending the back knee and looking at the wide, vast open yang sky.

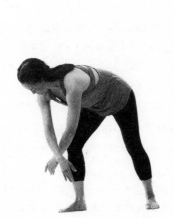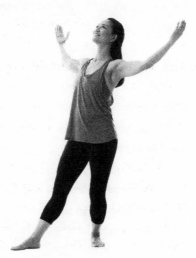

6. Continue, completing 5–7 rounds, and then change legs, stepping the right foot back in and the left foot forward.

7. Repeat Steps 2–5 on the second side, with the left foot stepping forward. Remember that when you are exhaling, the front knee bends, crossing the arms. When you are inhaling, the weight shifts and the arms continue to cross until they are overhead. The palms will be facing each other.

8. When you have completed the second side, step the front foot back into *Wuji*.

9. Do one round of the Closing Form for Peaceful Qi (see page 61): gather the energy of the sky around you with the hands, lifting them to the sides and then overhead. Once your hands are overhead, slowly turn them so that the palms face the earth. Moving your hands slowly down in front of your face, lungs and large intestine, use your hands to fill with the yang sky energy.

10. Finish by placing your hands stacked on the lower *dantian*. Observe how your body and breathing feel.

Shake the Back Seven Times to Eliminate the 100 Illnesses (*Bei Hou Qi Dian Bai Bing Xiao*)

This form is traditionally done as the last of the Eight Silk Brocades. In Chinese, the phrase '100 illnesses' (*bai bing*) means 'all kinds of diseases'. This form is believed to help eliminate general illness and disease. The gentle shaking done in this practice is said to help settle the qi. It is believed to help condition the lungs by improving blood circulation and aiding recovery from fatigue. It also benefits the liver and the Water organs of the kidneys and urinary bladder. Generally, it is described as making your body and spirit feel refreshed, renewed and revitalised.

FORM INSTRUCTIONS

1. From *Wuji* (picking up from the last form), take a few long, slow, even, fine and deep breaths.

2. Exhale and roll the head forwards and down, bending all the way down into a comfortable forward fold. Keep the knees bent.

3. Inhale and roll all the way up and back into an easy backbend. Let your hips move forwards and arms release back behind you.

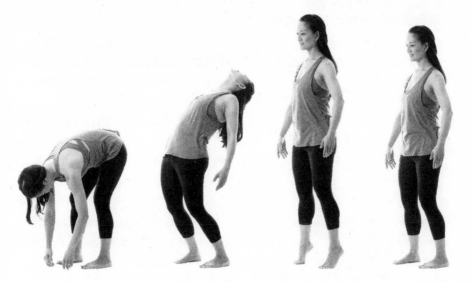

4. Exhale and lift your torso back into centre. Lift and drop your heels down, so that you gently shake the back. It will feel like a gentle bounce.

5. Continue, rolling forward with your exhale, and rolling up and back with your inhale. Be cautious not to overextend the lower back in either your forward fold or backward bend. The backbend should feel mild – remember, the definition of mild will vary for each individual.

6. When you exhale and come up, shake gently.

7. Continue, repeating for 7 rounds to eliminate the 100 illnesses.

8. When you finish, stand in *Wuji*.

9. Complete one round of the Closing Form for Peaceful Qi (see page 61). Begin to gather healthy qi in your palms as they reach to the sides and overhead. Once the hands are overhead, turn the palms to face the earth and fill with healthy qi that supports eliminating tiredness, fatigue and the 100 illnesses.

10. Finish by placing your hands stacked on your lower *dantian*, observing how your body, mind and spirit feel.

CHAPTER 20

Grief and Appreciation:
The Emotion and Spirit of Metal

Whether it be the loss of summer's warm, bright days, the end of a romance or losing a loved one, each of us experiences grief. Grief is the emotion related to Metal. When we grieve, we mourn for something that has passed. For most people, losing someone or something we cherish can be crushing. It is certainly not as easy as acquiring something we desire, or otherwise gaining in some way. Denying grief is common. It is a subject most people tend to avoid because it is an emotion that is often too painful to bear. Many may also feel wary of showing their grief, because it risks exposing frailty or weakness. We would rather control our feelings than let them show our potential vulnerability.

I remember after my father passed away, I was shocked that no one from Beijing reached out to console my mother – not even the general manager of my father's company or their closest friends. I remember feeling angry and confused about the silence. She was in California at the time, but to me, this did not excuse their silence. I was convinced that perhaps the grief of someone dying, like many painful emotions in China, was too much, and perhaps something people chose to ignore or push away.

I was wrong. The day my mother returned to Beijing, the outpouring of visitors started. People who had known my father for years or decades began to come to pay their respects. As it turned out, grief was not something one could express through a text, email or phone call. For Chinese of my parents' generation, grief had to be done in person. The friends who came to visit my mother spent hours at our house, often in tears. They bowed to my father's altar, lit incense and recalled stories. For each person, paying a visit was an opportunity to express and release their sadness. Their company was also a gift to my mother: with so many visitors, she was rarely alone. She was also reminded daily that so many people loved and respected my father.

In Chinese medicine and qigong, grief and loss are part of the natural life cycle of growth and decay. As such, it is a valid emotion that we can learn to work with and honour, which lets us see that which is treasured and of most essence in our lives. We can begin to see that letting go also opens us up to new forms of connection and appreciation. For my family, losing my father was devastating, but through our loss we also grew closer and more connected than we had been in years.

When we open to the pain of grief in a balanced way, we can also begin to increase our wherewithal to meet difficulty with grace. When we are able to accept loss and move through it, we have the opportunity to become more resilient and capable of moving through life with greater determination and purpose. Grief has the capacity to awaken Metal's characteristics of strength, courage and dignity. We may also start to feel closer to spirit and move beyond our material existence. With my father, for example, while I knew that he was physically gone, I began to feel his spirit and love eternally present within me as well as all around me.

Grief enables us to remember that something of immense meaning and value remains with us despite our loss. When we lose those we love, we can be reminded that our time on this earth is precious. Their passing can make us appreciate the limited time we have to live and value moments with loved ones more fully.

Imbalanced grief, however, can express as denial. If we push grief away or avoid it altogether, we run the risk of not only stifling our loss but also stifling and dissociating from our other emotions and experiences such as love, happiness and creativity. This can lead to a deep tension within ourselves. When we feel tense, we tend to close down and become less responsive to life. This impacts our mental and physical health, but may also unintentionally alienate and hurt those we love.

We can also have too much grief. The pain of losing someone we love stems from loving them so much and missing them dearly. We cannot imagine life without them. Like digestion, however, grief is a process that we move through and moves through us. If we can allow it to happen and summon the courage to accept our pain and heartache, in time our body, mind and spirit can process grief and eventually learn to let go and move on.

When we cannot let go, we carry our grief and it weighs us down. Too much grief depresses and burdens the lungs. When we are grief-stricken, we can often find breathing more difficult. When we cannot let go of the past, we have a hard time opening up to and appreciating our present lives.

Grief allows appreciation for life

In many ways, appreciation can be understood as the virtue and spirit of Metal. Often, we only appreciate something when we are about to lose it or after it has gone. With Metal in qigong and Chinese elements, however, we can begin to acknowledge what we have before it is lost. Appreciation is being present and seeing the beauty of changing colours in the autumn leaves, a conversation with a friend, or something as ordinary yet also extraordinary as a single breath. Grief wakes us up and can give us strength and determination to make the most out of life. We develop the fierce courage to accept that all things change, and there is no better time than now to appreciate what we have.

Qigong helps us meet the emotional challenge of grief by learning how to honour what we have had and gracefully let go of what is ready to fall away. This helps us open to new possibility. At a physical level, we can learn to let go of what we cling to unconsciously, such as tension and rigidity in the body. When we let tension go, we make room for more spaciousness, flow and ease. In our efforts, we can let go of unnecessary sloppiness or crass movements, and orientate towards a deeper refinement and quality. In our emotions, we can also begin to let go.

Qigong Practices for Supporting Healthy Grief and Appreciation of Life

These three practices use very gentle movements that I have found can support the emotion of grief in ways that allow it to be felt while also reminding us of how to appreciate and be inspired by life. The practices can be done sitting on a cushion or chair, or standing in *Wuji*. Each can be done from one minute up to five minutes each.

METAL ORGAN AND ELEMENT MUDRAS

This is part of the Five Element Mudra practices, and can be done on its own or in conjunction with the other elemental mudras. It involves a series of hand positions that are simple yet highly effective in supporting our ability to process and work with grief in skilful ways. Because grief is generally a difficult and delicate emotion that can easily be pushed away or hidden, this practice gently addresses grief and works with it implicitly rather than directly, by supporting and nourishing the lungs, which are believed to store grief. The movements invite us to soften and gently let go, while also opening to appreciation and new possibilities.

Each movement flows from one to the next. It is a relaxing yet powerful set of movements that are believed to help Metal come into harmony and balance.

Holding the Moon at the Chest

FORM INSTRUCTIONS

1. Start sitting comfortably on a chair or cushion, or standing in *Wuji*. Take a few long, slow, even, fine and deep breaths.

2. Inhale and lift the hands, with the palms turned away from the body to the level of the chest. Imagine you could shape your hands around a full moon. The thumbs point towards each other without touching, and the other four fingers of each hand remain at a 45-degree angle, facing each other, without touching. The thumbs are set apart from the index, middle fingers, ring and pinkie fingers.

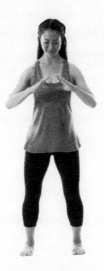

3. With the image of the moon, imagine its cyclical nature of waxing and waning, appearing and disappearing in the sky.

4. As you remain here for a few breaths (5–9 rounds), fine-tune the hand and arm position. Relax the thumbs. Allow the index fingers to be more active while you intentionally relax the middle, ring and pinkie fingers. Also, keep the elbows very soft, joints of the shoulders soft and the breath steady.

Hands Breathing Lungs

FORM INSTRUCTIONS

1. From Holding the Moon at the Chest, inhale and expand the arms and hands out to the sides, keeping them at shoulder height. The elbows should stay slightly bent, and the hands within your peripheral view.

2. Exhale, bring the arms back inwards, and begin to cross the wrists so that each hand is placed a few centimetres/inches in front of each lung. It does not matter which wrist is in front.

3. Inhale and imagine the hands can expand the energy of your lungs breathing in air. Simultaneously move your two hands a few centimetres/inches away from your chest with the wrists still crossed to allow for the expansion of the lungs. Imagine inspiration and energy filling your lungs.

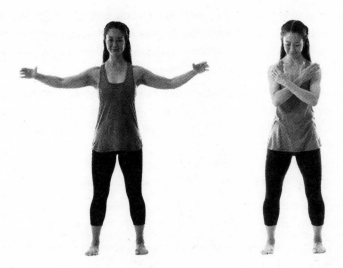

4. Exhale and imagine the hands can support the energy of your lungs breathing out air. Simultaneously move your two hands back in towards your lungs without touching your skin, allowing for the contraction of the lungs. Imagine a soft, soothing quality that calms your two lungs.

5. Continue, allowing each movement and breath to be intentional, long, deep and smooth. Also let the movements of the hands be smooth and gradual.

6. Repeat for at least 9 rounds. You can continue to do this movement pattern for 3–5 minutes.

Hands Help with Letting Go

FORM INSTRUCTIONS

1. From Hands Breathing Lungs, inhale and expand the arms and hands out to the sides, keeping them at shoulder height. The elbows should stay slightly bent, and the hands within your peripheral view.

2. Exhale and take both hands behind you to your lower back. Gently hold each palm and hand on the opposite forearm. Rest the wrists, hands and forearms gently on the back body, where the bottom of your lungs are located, as well as the transverse colon. This area corresponds to the deeper capacity for the lungs to take in qi and inspiration, and the large intestine's ability to help us let go.

3. Inhale and feel your breathing concentrated to the area where your hands rest on your lower back. Exhale and feel your breathing release from this area. You may also choose to inhale appreciation, and exhale unnecessary holding on or grief.

4. Inhale and bring the hands to the front of your lower abdomen, palms turned away from each other and the backs of the hands turned towards each other. Let the fingers point towards the earth like the tentacles of a jellyfish. Keep the hands a few centimetres/inches apart so that the backs of the hands do not touch. Take a few breaths here – 5–9 or more – imagining unnecessary holding or tension can drip down off your fingertips.

5. To release, inhale and bend your elbows slightly back to your sides, palms facing the earth. Exhale and release the hands down by your sides.

6. To finish, place your hands stacked over the lower *dantian* and observe how you feel.

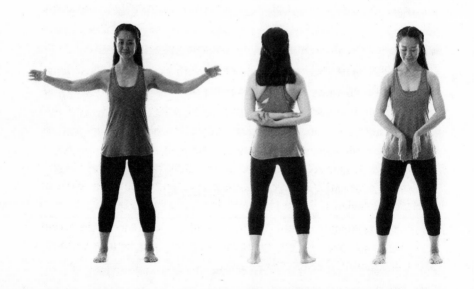

Closing Form for Peaceful Qi
(An Zhang Ping Qi)

As the previous elemental closing forms (see pages 61, 105 and 143), this clearing, gathering, sealing practice for Metal uses intention and simple movements to affect the emotions and movement of qi through the body.

FORM INSTRUCTIONS

1. Start in *Wuji*, taking long, slow, even, fine and deep breaths.

2. Breathe naturally and with awareness in the *dantian*. Continue this *dantian* breathing throughout the following movements.

3. Turn the palms out and begin to move them slowly and deliberately to the sides and then overhead. As you do this, gather the quality that may apply to you: rigidity or unnecessary holding on – the inability to grieve and accept loss; dullness or lack of enthusiasm – the inability to appreciate life.

4. Once the hands are overhead, turn the palms to face the earth, middle fingers pointing towards each other, elbows bent.

5. Slowly and deliberately begin to lower the hands down in front of your face, neck, chest and belly. Use the intention to clear out all you have just gathered.

6. The movement in Steps 3–5 then repeats, with a different intention: gather the gentle acceptance of loss, which is also a tremendous source of strength and courage; or gather appreciation or inspiration. These are qualities of grief when in balance. Fill these into the space you have cleared.

7. The final movement is to gather all you have filled: acceptance, appreciation and inspiration. Seal this into your roots to help you nourish balanced Metal in the form of your body.

FINAL NOTE

Once you have finished all three movements, remain in *Wuji* for a few breaths and absorb the way you feel. You can complete this by placing your palms on the lower *dantian* and noticing how you feel.

PART 5

Water Element

Nourishing Our Deepest Wisdom

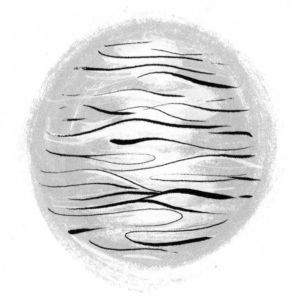

CHAPTER 21

Maximum Yin:
Water and Winter's Time to Rest

In Chinese medicine and qigong, winter is when Mother Nature lies fallow. It is a time of year when energy is conserved rather than expended. In the winter, many animals become less active or even dormant, and most plants store up resources through their root systems to see them through the next growth cycle. Most people today, however, are expected to be productive throughout the year. Rarely do we slow down and do less during winter. This is in part due to the near-constant demand from our jobs and society to be busy and contribute as much as we can, 100 per cent of the time. Yet, if we look to nature, busyness happens in cycles that usually follow intervals of rest. Qigong begins to help us honour these periods of rest in our daily and seasonal cycles. It also helps us respect the idea that as we mature into older age, rest is not a shortcoming; rather, it nourishes our capacity to listen and nourish our deeper wisdom. We will look at these ideas more in Chapters 23 and 25.

Seasonally, winter is a time of maximum yin, when daylight hours are shortest, temperatures coldest and movement more still. As microcosms of the macrocosm, human beings also require stillness and periods of rest that help us balance our energies. Our organs need time to rest, as does each of our cells. If we try to be productive all the time, we risk harming our organs and physically running out of resources. In a daily cycle, stillness and winter are the hours when we rest and sleep. Scientists still do not understand why we sleep, but some research suggests it is because our brains need to be repaired and cleared of waste.[1] Just as when we sleep and store up energy to move through a day, winter is when we can recover from our year before spring begins.

Water in the Chinese Five Element theory

Water is the fifth stage of the *wuxin*, or Five Phases and Elements. Rather than the upward maturity of growth created by heat and warmth, Water's cooling qualities create downward flow and inward attention. In the cyclical phases, Water controls Fire and puts out flames that burn too hot. It follows Metal in the creative cycle and is enriched by Metal's minerals. It comes before Wood, and nourishes and feeds the growth of grasses, plants and trees. It is also controlled by Earth, which blocks its tendency to overflow by creating banks, pools and dams.

Water in nature can manifest as oceans, rivers, streams, lakes, ponds and marshes. It is also the clouds, rain, snow and frost. In balance, qigong suggests we adapt our bodies, which are mostly fluid, to be more malleable and changeable like water. We will look at the aspects of fluidity in our bodies and how they relate to qigong in the next chapter on Water's effortless strength.

Water is life's true and unique medium. We live in the watery womb of our mother's uterus until we are born. As we age and grow, we rely on water for continued healthy development, especially at our cellular level.[2] For plants and flowers, water is a structural agent that enables them to take shape and reach towards the sun. Without water, life simply cannot be sustained.

In religions and myths, water also holds potent powers associated with creation, destruction and renewal. From Christian and Hebrew notions that God separated the waters to enable the world to emerge,[3] to ancient India's hymns of the *Rgveda* that describe how the world was brought into existence from Cosmic Waters.[4] Water generates life. Conversely, this life can also be taken away and relates to death. It is the River Ganges where many Hindus in India choose to go for cremation. It is the River Styx that, once crossed, leads to the land of the dead in Greek mythology. It is the flood sent as God's punishment to sinners that spared only Noah and those he could take on his ark.[5] Fountains of life and baptisms that purify the soul point to water's ability to revive and give new life. In Daoism, water is closely associated with the Dao itself: it is the source and origin of all things, powerful yet humble, nameless and shapeless yet that which ultimately nurtures and guides all life.

In balance, water flows effortlessly, like a gently moving mountain brook. This idea supports one of qigong's fundamental principles, known as *wuwei*. *Wuwei* means doing not-doing, effortless effort, action and non-action. It is the lynchpin of Daoist thought and the goal of seasoned qigong practitioners, martial artists and Daoist spiritual seekers. To experience *wuwei*, we can begin by perceiving and embodying the quality of Water in balance, which flows naturally and spontaneously in nature. We can also begin to notice when our Water falls out of balance. Sometimes our Water element can feel stagnant, sluggish and unable to flow – like the murky waters of a marsh. Other times, it may be raging, as if it wants to overflow and flood the land. With qigong, we begin to orientate our intentions and practice towards the balanced, free flow of water. We will look at how we can do this in more detail in the next chapter.

As qigong draws heavily from Daoist ideas and views of the world, many of the movements and practices naturally help to balance our Water element, which is like the Dao itself. This balance, like all the elements we have explored, happens at the level of our body, mind, emotions and spirit.

The following chapters will look at how qigong best supports this balance through a combination of context and practice.

CHAPTER 22

Water's Soft Strength

As the *Dao De Jing* describes, 'Nothing in the world is as soft and yielding as water, yet for dissolving the hard and inflexible, nothing can surpass it'.[6] In nature, water can indeed be gentle and fluid, yet so powerful it carves the Grand Canyon. As an element, it can take the most jagged rock and eventually transform it into a polished, round stone. This metaphor can serve us well when practising qigong: when we move our bodies like water, we can adopt a soothing naturalism and flow. Over time, this aim begins to wear down the most persistent tension, discomfort and tiredness we hold in our bodies.

Fluidity in movement and life

With qigong, we begin to foster qualities of water's fluid, soft strength by imagining our movements ebb and flow in continuous and unbroken ways. As we move our arms and hands through forms, we can imagine that they float along currents of water that glide them from one position to the next. We can also begin to soften rather than tense or push against areas of the body that are tight. In Chinese, this ability is called *suihe*, or to 'flow the way the river flows'. When we practise moving with the idea of *suihe* in our bodies, our movements can take on the adaptable, shifting motion of rivers and streams. When we recall our body's fluid make-up (60–70 per cent of the body is fluid), we can ride the currents of sensations and begin to support an optimal relationship with our watery constitutions.

We can also learn to bring these qualities of fluidity into our daily life. Described by psychology as the 'flow state', we can apply understandings of Water's ability to flow naturally and spontaneously to help us feel 'in the zone', immersed and able to enjoy what we do. In qigong, this is equivalent to *wuwei*, or effortless effort. Think of a martial artist who is active and alert, yet also focused, quiet and inwardly composed, or firefighters who know precisely where to position themselves to extinguish a blaze. Regardless of the chaos, busyness or danger, their bodies and minds are clear. By cultivating fluidity of movement associated with the Water element, we foster our capacity for an inward stillness and calm, regardless of our circumstances.

WHERE THE FLUIDS OF THE BODY CAN BE FOUND

In the joints: as synovial fluid, which is like a dilatant fluid that lubricates between joint surfaces and helps with shock absorption.

In the bones: as citrate layers (gel), which is the primary load-bearing material in bone. Our bones are made of 50 per cent fluid from the citrate layers (gel).

In the veins, arteries, capillaries and heart: as blood that circulates. The heart circulates blood in a figure-of-8. As blood flows through the veins, arteries and capillaries, it moves with quite turbulent flow – like a whirlpool or fast-moving river.

Between the cells: as interstitial fluid, the extracellular fluid between our cells. We have 11 litres (19 pints) of this fluid (more than the blood in the body!). It functions to provide nutrients to our cells and transport waste.

Between the organs: as periorgan fluid, which helps lubricate and moisten surfaces of viscera, and softens between visceral structures of the organs. It is present in the inner skin of the chest and abdominal wall.

In the lungs: as pleural fluid, which serves to reduce friction during movements of respiration.

In the heart: as serous fluid that eliminates friction as the heart beats.

In the skull and spinal cord: as cranio-sacral fluid that cleans the central nervous system and drains hormones and antibodies. It is also a buffer that protects the tissue layers of the spinal cord and skull. It moves 2000 times slower than blood and takes 6–8 hours to make a full circuit.

In the lymphatic system: as lymphatic fluid. We move about 5 litres (9 pints) of lymph every day. The lymphatic system has no pump, but is 'pumped' by the movement of the diaphragm. It moves inward from the extremities and sits near capillaries. It follows our veins, except around our organs, and has a clear movement, unlike the whirlwind patterns of blood.

Wuwei *in qigong*

The notion of action/non-action can seem counterintuitive to many people. This is because most of the time, we associate actively doing things – for example, deeply stretching into a part of the body to release tightness – as being better than leaving it alone. While some stretching certainly helps and some discipline is necessary to work skilfully with our bodies, with qigong, each of our efforts ideally points us towards the goal of effortlessness; we only use as much action as is necessary to achieve an outcome, nothing more.

When we are relaxed, free and focused, we feel *wuwei* naturally arise. It is the antithesis of strife and struggle. When we practise qigong and begin to relax places we normally tighten, such as in the hands, jaw and face, we begin to do what water does naturally: gradually dissolve the hard and inflexible. In time, and with practice, qigong allows us to enter into an even and unbroken flow.

Wuwei is a state that can only be cultivated rather than practised. How do we cultivate *wuwei*? A good place to start is by embracing the qualities of Water's soft strength and fluid ease when we practise qigong.

Practices to Nourish Water's Soft Strength

This series of three qigong forms helps connect us to the soft strength of water. The first two, Moving Clouds and Pushing Waves, can also be done as part of the 18 Forms, and the last practice, Rippling Waves, can be included as part of the Five Element Mudras. Each can also be done on its own. The forms also integrate imagery that enables us to feel a direct relationship to nature: we move clouds, push waves and ripple our hands on the surface of water. When we connect to water as it exists in nature, we can begin to feel the natural fluidity that is within us, as well as all around us.

Moving Clouds
(*Ma Bu Yun Shou*)

This form applies the image of using your hands to move imaginary clouds between them. The visualisation guiding the movement encourages a smoothness and suppleness that lends to the fluid movements of the body. Regular practice is believed to help soften and relax the fight/flight/freeze branch of our nervous system, introducing a more easeful yet awake energetic state in the body.

Moving Clouds is also part of the 18 Forms. It is the tenth form in the series. The direct translation from Chinese is 'Cloud Hands in Horse Stance'. I believe Moving Clouds evokes a similar notion but also asks the hands to become soft, strong agents that are capable of doing something etheric, such as move cloud matter, naturally and effortlessly between them.

FORM INSTRUCTIONS

1. Start in *Wuji*, taking long, slow, even, fine and deep breaths.
2. Step the feet slightly wider apart into an easy Horse Stance.
3. Bring your hands towards your centre, right hand above left, with the palms facing each other. Keep the hands separated by 30–40 cm (12–16 inches). Imagine that your hands are holding clouds.

4. Inhale and begin to imagine moving clouds between your hands towards the right, turning your waist gently. Imagine the hands move soft, invisible cloud matter between them, naturally and effortlessly. As you move the clouds, let the lower hand stay at the level of the lower *dantian*. The upper hand can move at the level of the chest.

5. Once turned to a comfortable degree, switch the position of your hands by smoothly rolling your right hand down as you bring your left hand above, palms facing again.

6. Move the clouds between your hands smoothly towards the left, turning your waist gently. Again, imagine light, pillow-like cloud matter moving between them. Keep your hands soft and your body like the movement of water in a stream – supple, unbroken and calm.

7. To finish, bring the hands back towards your centre and turn them so that your thumbs are towards the sky and the palms face each other. Imagine holding a round cloud ball between them. Gently release the hands, palms facing down, releasing the hands that moved clouds.

8. Step back into *Wuji* and observe how you feel.

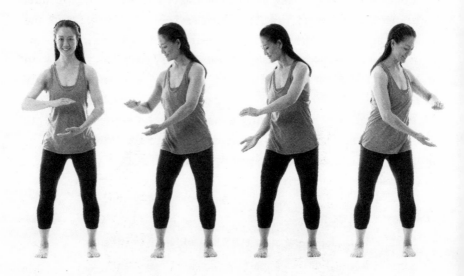

Pushing Waves
(*Tui Bo Zhu Lang*)

This form is part of the Tai Chi Qigong 18 Forms. Traditionally it is done as the twelfth form, but I like to do it as the thirteenth. Practice of this form helps create ease, grace and strength in the body. The movements involve visualising pushing an ocean wave, which is poetic and also impossible: we cannot push a wave. Yet when doing the practice, the movements seem familiar. As waves gently crest, we can conjure the soft, subtle strength it would take to push something formless like water. Paradoxically, when I do this form I also feel the effortlessness and ease of *wuwei*. Rather than push the waves, I harmonise with them and rock forwards and backwards in gentle ebbs and flows.

FORM INSTRUCTIONS

1. Start in *Wuji*, taking long, slow, even, fine and deep breaths.

2. Step your right foot forward and slightly to the right into a short Bow Stance. The feet should be at least shoulder-distance wide. You should be able to comfortably bend your front and back knee. When doing this form, the weight alternately shifts forwards and back between the front and back legs.

3. While bending the front knee, exhale and push the hands away from your chest as if pushing an ocean wave. You can also use the back foot to push away.

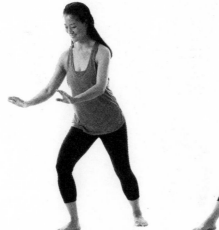
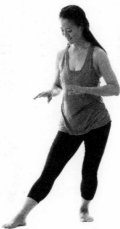

4. Inhale and retract the hands, softening them back in, as if pulling a wave towards you. Do this while also bending the back knee. Your weight will be primarily on the back leg and foot.

5. Exhale, and repeat this movement of pushing waves for 6–9 rounds.

6. When you finish, step the right foot in and prepare to change sides.

7. Step the left foot forwards and repeat Steps 3–5 for 6–9 rounds.

8. When you finish, step the left foot back into *Wuji*. Either end the practice here and observe how your breathing and body feel, or continue to the next form.

Rippling Waves Water Mudra

This form is one of the Five Element Mudras and is a simple yet powerful movement involving the hands. It involves imagining the arms and hands rippling like the movement of water on the top of a gently moving stream. This movement evokes Water's unbroken and spontaneous tendencies. As the arms ripple in and out, the legs also alternately bend and straighten, creating a gentle pulse up and down.

FORM INSTRUCTIONS

1. Start in *Wuji*, taking long, slow, even, fine and deep breaths.

2. Inhale and gently bend your knees. At the same time, begin to ripple your arms gently forwards, like a ribbon. Let this movement be led primarily

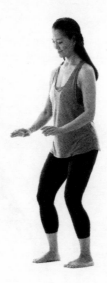

from your wrists. Let the arms lift to the level of the solar plexus. Gently let your tailbone lower while you keep your head upright. Keep your hands very relaxed as they move.

3. Exhale and straighten your legs slightly, lifting from the crown of your head. Simultaneously retract your arms and hands, letting them ripple in towards you as you lower them by your sides.

4. Continue for 9–15 rounds, inviting a ribbon-like rippling movement to remain moving in continuous and unbroken rhythms, with your breath and body gently rising and lowering.

5. Finish with an exhale to release the arms in and down by your sides. Then inhale, bending your elbows slightly back. Exhale and release your palms turned towards the earth, as though the hands themselves are resting on the surface of the water.

6. Stand in *Wuji* and observe how the body feels.

7. After a moment or two, do the Closing Form for Peaceful Qi (see page 61): gather the hands to the sides, lift them slowly overhead and then lower them, palms facing the earth in front of your face, chest and belly. Place your hands on your lower *dantian*. Breathe.

CHAPTER 23

Water's Deep Listening and Stillness

The ability to truly listen is a quality of healthy, balanced Water in qigong and Chinese medicine. Each element has an associated sense organ and for Water, this is the ear. When our hearing is impaired, this can sometimes be a sign that we have a Water imbalance. Yet the ability to listen extends beyond our ability to hear.

聽

To understand the richness of listening, we can look at the meaning of 'to listen' in Chinese. The original, complex character for 'to listen' is a compound of two characters: the ear and virtue. The character for the ear also has beneath it the radical for a person standing to give their attention. The character for virtue includes the radicals for the heart, the eye and undivided attention.[7] Thus, when we listen, we do far more than decipher what someone says; we become present and bring forth our heart. When we listen, we do what the German philosopher Paul Tillich described as our first responsibility of love, which is to listen.[8]

How can we learn to better listen in our lives? With qigong, we begin by becoming more closely attuned to our bodies and breath. We respect our energies throughout a day. We open to and align with the seasons as they change and affect us. We learn to honour our age and life experience. These are qualities that naturally develop in us when we embrace Water and its close association with the ability to slow down, become more still and listen deeply. To listen deeply and sincerely also means we cannot be talking or constantly filling our days with noise.

Listening requires the support of silence.

Stillness and silence

When our Water element is in balance, we can learn to appreciate silence. Silence supports deep listening. When practising qigong, it is often advised to practise as though you can listen to the sound of rain. To do this, we need quiet space. This is perhaps why many spiritual seekers, from Buddhist meditators to Quakers and Catholics, champion silence as necessary for deepening a connection to truth or God. Silence is also a fixture of nature. Qigong points us in this direction and reminds us that as part of the natural world, we can benefit from having the space and time to be silent, still and tranquil.

As with all qualities, however, stillness and silence can be balanced or imbalanced. The tendency with Water is to feel either stuck or hyperactive – two characteristics of Water out of balance. Qigong helps us find a balance between these states, so that we become calm and able to reflect everything around us, like a mountain lake. When we practise qigong, we begin to work to direct our body, mind and spirit towards the right amount of stillness, so that our lives feel fluid and calm, yet also full of depth, reserve and great potential. In this state we can perhaps tap into the Great Source of Nature, or the Oneness of the Dao.

Practices for Water's Stillness and Deep Listening

The following two meditations can help create and maintain a sense of deep peace and stillness. The first meditation is called Embryonic Breathing. There are countless approaches to practising this breathing technique that have been described over the centuries. While detailed books have been written about this breathing technique, I have chosen a basic approach to begin practising it safely and effectively. The second meditation uses three points in acupuncture for a visualisation practice that is calming and helps to remind us of Water's source of quietness, as well as potential to support life.

You can do these practices sitting on a chair or cushion, or lying down on your back. If you choose to sit, sit with your back upright. If you lie down, you may wish to place a pillow under your head and a rolled towel, blanket or yoga bolster under your knees, for comfort.

Embryonic Breathing
(*Tai Xi*)

This practice moves through four preparatory stages of breathing before starting embryonic breath. Embryonic breathing is a peaceful and natural breath that we hardly know happens. Some see it as similar to cellular respiration, which is how cells in our body breathe. It is also how we breathed in utero.

> You may wish to do this with your eyes closed. If you are lying down it can be easy to fall asleep, so you may wish to keep one hand raised so that the forearm is perpendicular to the ground. This will provide enough awareness and presence to stop you dozing off.

FORM INSTRUCTIONS

1. **Deep breathing:** Breathe deeply into the whole body, inhaling through the nose and exhaling through the mouth. Feel the breath move as fully through the body as you can. Repeat for 6–9 rounds.

2. **External breathing:** Inhale breath and qi into the middle *dantian*, which is the area of your solar plexus and chest. Exhale and descend the breath you bring in to the lower *dantian*, or area of your abdomen. Imagine that the breath brings in vital, nourishing qi that also descends to the lower *dantian*, and exhales toxic qi as you breathe out. This type of breathing is performed in a way sometimes known as 'reverse breathing', or *ni hu xi*. As you breathe in, the abdomen deflates while the chest inflates. As you breathe out, the abdomen inflates and the chest deflates. Repeat for 6–9 rounds.

3. **Internal breathing:** This breathing is also sometimes called Mingling Sun and Sea, or Fire and Water. This is the opposite of external or reverse breathing. Visualise the lower *dantian* as the ocean or sea. Then, visualise the middle *dantian* as the sun. Imagine pure breath and clean, vital qi already in the body. Inhale this qi from the middle *dantian* to the lower *dantian*, as though the sun might shine its warmth downward to warm the

cool oceans. Exhale and let this rise back up from the lower *dantian* to the middle *dantian*, as though the cool waters of the ocean might cool the heat of the sun. Repeat 6–9 rounds of breath and visualisation of this movement and exchange.

4. ***Dantian* breathing:** With this practice, let the breath and qi remain concentrated in the lower *dantian*. Let the breath rise and fall from the *dantian*, as if nourishing the waters of your deepest reservoirs, ensuring they are replenished and full. There is no need to count the number of rounds, simply use this breath for 2–5 minutes (or as long as is comfortable without becoming drowsy or dull).

5. **Embryonic breathing:** With this last stage, we enter into an effortless breathing that is slow and natural. Simply let the body breathe. It may be like you are unaware that you are breathing, yet it happens autonomously and gently. You may feel as though you become the breath and become the *qi*. Breathe as long as is comfortable, for 3–10 minutes.

6. Either proceed from here to the next breathing exercise of the Three Stars of the *Dantian* or finish by gently bringing yourself back into the room by opening the eyes, if they were closed. Notice how you feel.

Three Stars of the *Dantian* (*Dantian San Xin*)

This practice is based on a meditation described in Ronald Davis's book, *Qigong Through the Seasons*.[9] Whenever I have practised or shared this with students, the feeling of stillness is palpable. It utilises three acupuncture points as focuses for attention. One of these points was introduced in Chapter 12 on Earth and intention (see page 115): Meeting of Yin (*Hui Yin*), at the base of the pelvic floor. A second point is called the Sea of Qi (*Qi Hai*), located on the abdomen a few centimetres/ inches below the navel, and a third point is called Gate of Life (*Ming Men*). This point is on the lower back between the second and third lumbar vertebrae, directly behind from the Sea of Qi. Gate of Life is on the yang Governing Channel, or *Du Mai*. As a yang point, it helps warm the body, like the light of the sun. It brings new energy and life to our experiences, and is especially nourishing for the kidneys – the yin organs associated with the Water element.

By doing this practice, we create a basin or pool in our lower *dantian*, abdomen and pelvis. This can become a source of qi, like a reservoir from which we can draw energy to nourish and sustain life. We also begin to warm this reservoir from Gate of Life on the lower back, like the sun rising over the ocean waters.

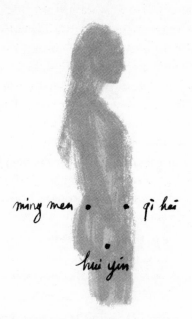

ming men · · qi hai

hui yin

The practice can be done on its own, or after Embryonic Breath. This can be a short meditation of 10–12 minutes, or a longer one lasting for 20–25 minutes.

VISUALISATION INSTRUCTIONS

1. Visualise Sea of Qi on the abdomen, a few centimetres/inches beneath the navel, as a calm, tranquil body of water, with gentle waves rippling on the surface. Breathe in and out at the Sea of Qi point. Concentrate on this point for 2–5 minutes.

2. Visualise Meeting of Yin, at the base of the pelvic floor. Breathe into this point. Breathe out and let the still surface of the Sea of Qi drop down towards Meeting of Yin, at the bottom of the pelvic floor, like a tideline descending. As you continue to breathe, invite the energy of the body to flow and settle downwards to this area. Concentrate on nourishing stillness and depth through the downward-settling qi for 2–5 minutes.

3. Then begin to visualise the movement of energy upwards, from Meeting of Yin to Gate of Life. Gate of Life is a strong source of yang energy. Breathe in and imagine energy moving from Meeting of Yin rising to Gate of Life. Exhale and invite Gate of Life to grow warmer and brighter, like the golden light of the sun. This image will begin to gently heat the contents of your lower *dantian*. Concentrate on inhaling from Meeting of Yin to Gate of Life, and exhaling to warm Gate of Life, for 2–5 minutes.

4. Start to bring the warmed Gate of Life qi forward towards Sea of Qi. Inhale into Gate of Life. Exhale and shine the light forward, like the light of the sun rising over the ocean to awaken new life and possibility. Maintain this breathing pattern and visualisation for 2–5 minutes.

5. Finish by letting the visualisations and specific points for breathing go. Place your hands stacked over the lower *dantian*. Notice your breathing and observe how the mind, body and spirit feel.

CHAPTER 24

Water's Organs:
The Kidneys and Urinary Bladder

The kidneys in Chinese medicine also pair with the urinary bladder as the organs and meridians associated with winter. Together, they help regulate how we use energy throughout a day, as well as a lifetime. The amount of energy we have available is determined by *jing*, or essence, which is stored in our kidneys.

Jing – *original essence*

Jing is a dense form of qi that affects our entire energy and make-up. There are two types of *jing*. The first type is given to us at birth, called prenatal *jing*. It is our original qi, or *yuan qi*. This original qi is believed to be passed down by our parents at birth and stored in our kidneys. As a congenital energy, it determines our basic constitution, such as our health, strength and appearance. How much *jing* we inherit can depend on our mother's health, diet and lifestyle during pregnancy, which in turn was determined by her mother's pregnant constitution. We are only given so much prenatal *jing* in life. Once it is used up, it is gone. Because of demanding and stressful lifestyles, many of us tend to deplete our *jing* prematurely. This is believed to lead to problems such as loss of libido, hearing, greying hair or a shorter lifespan.

The second type of *jing* is that which we acquire in life. This is postnatal *jing*. This type of *jing* can be affected by diet, meditation, exercise and lifestyle. Qigong, and practices like tai chi chuan and internal alchemy (neigong), focus on building healthy postnatal *jing* while simultaneously slowing down the loss of prenatal *jing*. For centuries, Daoists also held the view that through certain breathing, dietary and alchemical processes, human beings could restore our prenatal *jing* and attain immortality.[10]

Both types of *jing* influence the way we develop, and both are believed to affect our energy levels and reproductive health. Understanding how qigong practices affect our *jing* can be valuable and immediately useful. Not only can we use our practice to help us have more control over our energy, but we can also potentially stave off the negative effects of ageing. Since *jing* resides in the kidneys, a closer look at how we can work with our kidneys and their paired organ of the urinary bladder will lend support to the ways we can nourish our foundational and source energies.

The Kidneys

The kidneys filter approximately 180 litres (317 pints) of nourishment and waste every day. The waste filtered out is released by our bladder as urea and uric acid, and the nourishment filtered in is water that is reabsorbed into the bloodstream. The kidneys also help regulate our blood pressure and ensure our pH levels do not become too acidic or alkaline. Their bean-like shapes sit either side of our spine, at the junction of our mid and lower back. In Western medicine, we need our kidneys to live. Without them, we would die within minutes unless we underwent kidney dialysis. As such, they are the yin organ in Chinese medicine – the organs without which we cannot live.

In addition to storing our *jing*, the kidneys in Chinese medicine and qigong are the source of our primary yin and yang energies. As such, they are considered the foundations of life. They help us regulate our energy and baseline warmth. When the kidneys are weak, it is believed that our ability to live fully is negatively affected.[11] We can physically feel withdrawn, suffer from reproductive complications and an overall lack of vitality. When healthy, we feel a calm, quiet strength and reserve. The kidneys also have other practical functions. They are believed to preside over the health of our body's bones and teeth, affect the thickness of our hair, drive our will, govern our fear and determine our sexual urges and reproductive health. They affect our hearing, energy levels, refine and store the qi from our lungs and are connected to the Gate of Life acupuncture point that can rekindle our life's Fire.[12]

The Chinese system of medicine groups the function of the kidneys with the adrenal glands, which sit directly above them. The adrenal glands are part of our endocrine system and produce important hormones and steroids, most notably adrenaline and cortisol. Cortisol is known as the 'stress hormone'. When cortisol levels are too high, we can suffer from inflammation, stress, depression, mental illness and a lower life expectancy.[13] Adrenaline increases our heart rate and blood flow to our muscles. It is the main hormone that kicks in our fight/flight/freeze response, which is most commonly triggered by fear and stress. When our fears are in check, we can move through experiences that frighten us, and potentially grow and learn from them. As we shall see in the next chapter, fear is the emotion related to Water.

Urinary Bladder

Compared to the kidneys, the bladder has a far smaller role. It is located in front of the kidneys and is connected to them by ducts called the ureters. The bladder sac is small when empty, hollow and about the size of a pear. It can stretch, however, to quite a large size, and hold up to 2 litres (3½ pints) of fluid when full.

In Chinese medicine and qigong, the bladder is the yang organ of water. Its main function is to regulate the kidney's stored and transformed blood and qi. It transports nourishment from the kidneys and regulates our body's base temperature. It also eliminates anything filtered by the kidneys, through our urine.

Mentally and spiritually, the urinary bladder uses the kidney's will (*zhi*) and translates it into our ability to serve ourselves and others in kind and virtuous ways. When balanced, our bladder helps regulate how we store and utilise our energy, or qi reserves. It also ensures that the light of our *jing*, or inborn essence and potential, illuminates our lives. This illumination empowers us to see more clearly and develop a more accurate perception of reality. This in turn can grow into insight and deeper wisdom. One of my favourite points in acupuncture is the Bladder-One point, called 'Bright Eyes' (*Jing Ming*), located on the inner corner of the eye. I love this point because when I have it needled in acupuncture, I immediately feel my energy lift. Its main function is to help unite our inner and outer sources of light,[14] and encourage the radiance of our essence (*jing*) to shine forth – like sunlight dancing in the eyes of a child. Conversely, when out of balance, we may feel dim, or like there is no light to shine. We may also feel lethargic and lacking a drive or will do work or engage with others.

THE BLADDER AND KIDNEY MERIDIANS

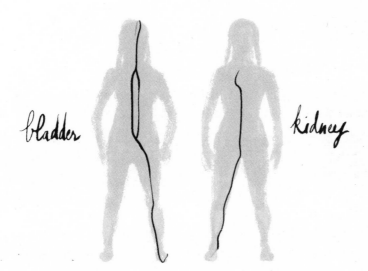

BLADDER

The bladder's key hours are from 3.00 to 5.00 p.m. This is the perfect time for an afternoon tea break, as liquid waste is released and some energy from the kidneys restored. As hours related to storage, it can be a good time to immerse in reading or light work.

The bladder meridians are some of the longest in the body. They run from the inner corner of the eye, around the head and down the two sides of the spine, where they continue down the back of the legs, knees, calves and ankles. They continue along the outer edge of each foot and end on the outer pinkie nail of the little toes.

KIDNEYS

The kidneys' hours are 5.00–7.00 p.m. As this is a time when we can connect to our primordial energies, it's a good time to begin to wind down our day and rest. Because the kidneys also store our postnatal essence (*jing*), it is a good time to feed our bones and have a nice meal.

The kidney meridian starts on the centre of the sole of each foot. From there, it moves up the sole of the foot and continues up through the inner ankles, calves, knees, thighs and groin. It then travels up both sides of the midline of the torso, and ends under the collarbone.

Practices to Nourish the
Kidneys and Urinary Bladder

The forms in this sequence can be an effective practice for building healthy kidney qi. They are each part of other sets of qigong practices, such as the Five Animal Frolics, Five Elements and 18 Forms, that work well together as a set. As such, you can do them as forms within those series, on their own, or in this sequence for the water organs. The practice takes about 10 minutes in total. It can help revive your energy while also calming the mind. For this reason, I think of this series as an ideal study break, especially in the late afternoon hours that relate to the urinary bladder and kidneys.

Bear Forms

The bear is the animal associated in qigong with winter. The forms, part of the Five Animal Frolics, draw on the power and strength of the bear, but also use twisting and rotational movements that directly stimulate and release tension from the area of the kidneys and adrenal glands. As determined creatures that move with heaviness, power and perseverance, bears conserve energy, yet know when and how to put their strength forward to achieve their goals. As you do these practices, you might invoke the heavy power of the bear. Also imagine that your qi weight sinks down to the lower *dantian*, which can help nourish the *jing* in the kidneys.

There are many Bear forms in qigong, and many interpretations of how to do the forms. I have chosen the two that I like to practise most, as they release tension in my back but also make me feel powerful and full of perseverance. These two forms build suppleness in the waist and strength through the legs and arms. They also warm the body, while nourishing and hydrating the muscles and joints.

BEAR TURNS

1. Start by standing in *Wuji*, taking long, slow, even, fine and deep breaths.
2. Step the feet wider apart for Horse Stance, with the knees bent.
3. Lift the hands and arms to shoulder height, bending the elbows at 90-degree angles. Keep the palms turned towards the sky, as if balancing platters on each hand.
4. Inhale. Then exhale and begin to turn your torso to the right. Keep the head lifted, spine upright and knees steady.
5. Inhale back to centre, keeping the hands as they are.

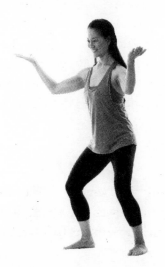 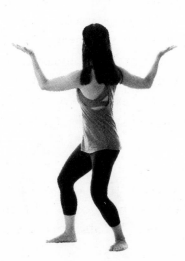

6. Exhale and turn your torso to the left. Again, keep the head lifted, spine upright and knees steady. This completes one round.

7. Continue, and repeat Steps 4–6 for 5–9 rounds. Emphasise the rotation of the spine and release through the lower back and kidneys.

8. To finish, inhale back to centre, keeping the hands up as though still holding platters, and begin the next Bear form.

BEAR PUSHES DOWN WITH TWO HANDS

1. From Bear Turns, exhale and turn to the right, but this time push both hands down, palms towards the earth. One hand will be in front of the abdomen and one behind the back. Imagine you are trying to push two fully inflated beach balls underneath the surface of water.

2. Inhale and turn back to centre, and lift the hands back to the starting position, with the hands holding imaginary platters.

3. Exhale and turn to the left, pushing both hands down, palms facing the earth, one hand in front of the abdomen and one hand behind the back.

4. Inhale back to centre again, lifting the hands back to shoulder height with the elbows bent. This completes one round.

5. Continue, repeating Steps 1–4 for 5–9 rounds. Emphasise the strength, power and downward movement of the hands.

6. After finishing 5–9 rounds, begin to release the hands.

7. Step the feet back into *Wuji*, observing how your breath, body and general energy levels feel.

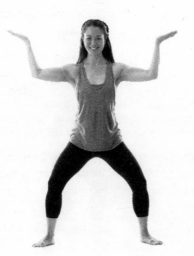 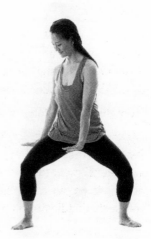

Turning the Flying Wheel
(*Huan Zhuan Fei Lun*)

This form is the sixteenth of the 18 Forms. It works to release tension in the back and turn the body from the centre and kidneys. The circular movement of the spine extending in all directions also stretches the urinary bladder lines that run along the two sides of the spine. It is deeply releasing, and a form that I have found helps replenish energy levels quickly.

Regular practice of this form helps purify the kidneys, urinary bladder, liver and intestines. It also circulates the blood flow more efficiently in the body, helping us eliminate waste materials and stagnation, and filling it with more vitality and space for the healthy, balanced flow of qi.

FORM INSTRUCTIONS

1. Start in *Wuji*, taking long, slow, even, fine and deep breaths.

2. Exhale and begin to fold forward, bending the knees comfortably. Keep the spine long and extended. Imagine the hands wrapping around the rim of a large wheel standing on its side.

3. Inhale and begin circling your imaginary wheel towards the right and overhead.

4. Exhale and circle the wheel down to the left and back towards the earth.

5. Continue, completing a total of three turns.

6. After three turns, reverse and turn the wheel towards the left, and turn it three times.

7. Once back in the forward-fold, flick your fingers towards the earth three times to flick off any additional waste or stagnation. As you flick all that is wasteful back to the earth, imagine it is compost that can be transformed by the earth as nourishment.

8. From the forward-fold, inhale and begin to rise back up to standing in *Wuji*.

9. Observe how you feel, and then do one round of the Closing Form for Peaceful Qi (see page 61). Inhale and gather vital essence from heaven, and nourishment for your blood and bones from the earth, in your hands as they reach out to the sides and then overhead. Turn the palms to face the earth, middle fingers pointing towards each other. Begin to lower the

hands down in front of your face, chest and torso, and fill with the qualities of healthy essence and energy to feed all aspects of your body, mind and spirit. At the same time, clear out any residual waste and toxicity, leaving your body clean, nourished and refreshed.

10. To finish, stand in *Wuji*, placing your hands stacked on the lower *dantian*, observing how you feel.

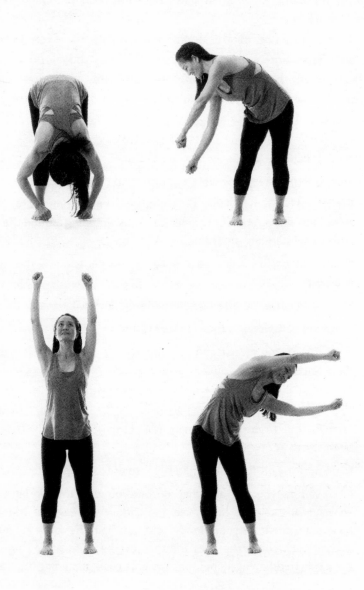

Five Element Water Practice

This form is part of the Five Element qigong practices. It uses the hands to trace along parts of the kidney as well as the urinary bladder lines of the legs. It taps the kidneys lightly to help stimulate their function and release tension that can feel tight around the lower back.

This form strengthens and helps to increase flexibility through the back, spine and legs. It also brings a pleasant warmth to the hands as they trace along the meridian lines that travel along the legs. With this practice, the sequence fosters the soft strength, deep listening and tenacity of Water in a fluid, natural way.

The form involves a gentle backbend and forward-fold. As such, it is important to modify this by bending the knees more deeply or taking a gentler backbend, especially if you have back injuries. As is true for any practice, if you have doubts, it is best to seek advice from a doctor before beginning to practise.

FORM INSTRUCTIONS

1. Start in *Wuji*, taking long, slow, even, fine and deep breaths. Then step the feet together.

2. Inhale, step the left foot out, knees bent, arms reaching out and backwards and then sweeping overhead into a gentle backward bend.

3. Exhale and fold forward. Remember to bend the knees and lengthen the spine, especially if your back feels tight.

4. Inhale and begin to trace your middle finger and hands up along the backs of your legs to your lower back. This is the urinary bladder meridian. It runs like a great river through the body, from the pinkie toes up through the backs of the legs and spine, all the way to the eyes.

5. Exhale, make soft fists with your hands and lightly tap your kidneys. When you tap, you stimulate *Ming Men* – or the Gate of Life.

6. Inhale and open the palms onto the kidneys.

7. Exhale and trace down the same lines of the back of the legs, your urinary bladder line.

8. Inhale your hands to the inner ankles and begin tracing the inner legs to the knees, thighs and groin. This is the kidney meridian.

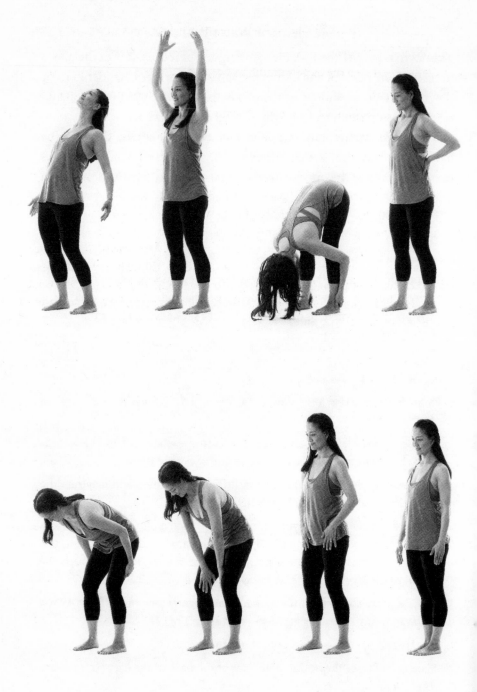

9. Exhale and release the hands, stepping the left foot back in, releasing the hands down.

10. Inhale and step the right foot out, and repeat Steps 2–8.

11. Exhale and release the hands, stepping the right foot next to the left, releasing the hands down. This completes one round.

12. Continue, and repeat Steps 2–11 with steady breathing. Complete 5–9 rounds.

13. After completing your 5–9 cycles, step back out into *Wuji* for the Closing Form for Peaceful Qi (see page 61): begin to extend the two hands to the sides and overhead. As you do this gather the qualities of your kidneys and urinary bladder in balance: balanced energy, hydrated, warm and full of vital essence. Then turn your palms to face the earth, moving the hands down in front of the face, chest and belly. Fill with these qualities. In the wake of these qualities filling into your body, you can also clear out imbalanced energy, weakness or a lack of will – aspects of the kidneys and urinary bladder that may arise when they are out of balance.

14. To finish, bring the hands in to rest on the lower *dantian*. Pause, noticing how the body feels.

CHAPTER 25

Fear, Will and Wisdom:
The Emotion and Spirit of Water

Freedom from fear has been a goal for many cultures, from ancient India to the modern world. The United Nations lists freedom from fear as one of the fundamental and universal human rights to which all people are entitled. In yoga and Buddhism, fearlessly seeing past misunderstandings and illusions, and a willingness to fully embrace life's inherent suffering, leads to freedom. In Daoism and qigong, when we align with and find harmony amidst the movements, patterns and rhythms of yin and yang, we understand that we are part of the Great Oneness of the tai chi axis. In this state, nothing is to be feared.

These aspirations and goals are noble, but for most people – certainly myself – fear is an emotion faced many times a day in overt and more subtle forms. Many of the subtle fears take the form of worries and concerns. Will I make it to teach my class in time? Will they like the food I've prepared? Is my mother OK living on her own? An overt fear may be while crossing the street on a busy road and hoping a car does not speed out from nowhere and hit me. Deeper fears, such as fear of who will care for me when I am older, or the fear of losing my loved ones if they travel to dangerous places or have been in an accident, also periodically surface.

A complete freedom from fear is an aspiration towards which I can work but am unlikely to fully reach in my lifetime. Still, I know that many times during or after a deep qigong practice, many of my subtle or deeper fears leave me. In the space of breathing, moving and feeling, I can be fully calm and present. In this state, I feel fearless.

When I consider the reasons for fearlessness arising in these moments, I can see that most of my fears are not realities; they are ideas and concepts in my mind that come and go like clouds, wind or rain. With qigong's emphasis on moving meditation, my body feels nourished and my mind less burdened. In this state, fears lose their grip on my mind and heart. I see how they arise and dissolve as part of the fluid, changing nature of all experience. I see them in their true form: present yet also impermanent. Qigong helps me remember that I am part of an ongoing and fluid process of change. When I feel this deeply, I begin to see that living my life fully also means releasing my fears and awakening more to my full potential to be alive and free.

In Chinese medicine, the ability to live fully and awaken to our full potential is governed by our *jing*, or essence. The primary obstacle to this potential, however, is fear – the emotion associated with Water in qigong and the Five Element framework. Like all emotions, fear can be balanced and imbalanced in our bodies and minds. Balanced fear is good fear: it helps us take action and find safety in dangerous situations. If we are walking alone at night and sense danger down a certain street, fear will turn us around or walk us down a different street. If houses are burning down our street, fear will tell us to leave before it's too late. But often we harbour fears that go beyond needing to stay safe. These are imbalanced fears that cause us to worry excessively and not be able to sleep at night. These can show up as anxieties, or undermining judgements against ourselves or others, that can, if left unchecked, become crippling to our physical, mental and emotional health.

Most of the time fear is an emotion that triggers unskilful responses. When we are afraid of something, we may act aggressively towards the object of our fear and lash out in some way. We may try to avoid our fear by running away from it, or somehow pushing it out of our mind. We can also feel frozen in our tracks when we are nervous or afraid, and not have a clue what to do. These tendencies are triggered by the nervous system that governs our fight/flight/freeze response, called the sympathetic nervous system.

As humans, we need this part of our nervous system to survive; without it, we would never do anything in the face of a perceived or real threat. Yet sometimes, we regard fear as a permanent truth rather than something that can – like all emotions and thoughts – shift and change. When we see fear as fixed, this overwhelms us and can prevent us from living up to our potential.

With qigong, the goal of working with fear is to support the body's natural ability to embrace a balanced attitude towards it. We do this by regular and consistent practice that begins to optimise the health of our Water organs, the kidney and urinary bladder. As we nurture the health of these organs, we may mitigate the fears that come when we feel energetically low or fatigued. We also begin to become more resilient and alert; we may be able to sense or even 'smell fear', which can help keep us physically safe. We also learn that, in certain situations, we can embrace the Water element's effortless strength and enhance our capacity to listen to ourselves and others. This helps us begin to see beneath the surface of our fears and look deeply into the origin of what frightens us. We learn to meet what is present with responsiveness rather than react aggressively, avoid or push it away.

Wisdom and will

We also begin to recognise that any true presence of fearlessness requires wisdom. If fearlessness is driven by adrenaline or ego, it can lead to acting thoughtlessly, irresponsibly or recklessly. If, however, fearlessness is born from a calm, steady and attentive place, then it can help us see the source of our unease or distress. Rather than being undone by fear, we see an opportunity to move past our struggles against fear and meet it with understanding and insight – qualities inherent in the reflective nature of Water. Insight helps us grow and learn from difficulty. When we meet our fears with the willingness to understand them more fully, we can begin to respond to life rather than constantly be caught up in cycles of reactivity. This enables us to nourish our deepest wisdom.

Ideally, Water's wisdom enables us to meet fear with resolve and purpose. In qigong and Chinese medicine, this resolve is our will, or *zhi*. *Zhi* speaks to our life's true purpose; it is an instinctual life force compelling us forward to act and achieve our life's volition. It is the product of *jing*, or essence, and the spirit of Water. The *zhi* that moves out from our essence is not wilful, but unfolds as a willingness to meet life and be responsive and fluid with its changing patterns and tides.

With healthy *zhi*, we begin to align our actions with our thoughts, speech and goals. We feel as though we know our purpose. We listen and respond to that which unnerves and challenges us with clarity and calm, rather than habitual reactivity or haste. Through this, we learn that we have the choice to meet fear and respond with love. We also feel as though we are connected to something greater than ourselves, whether this be nature, God or the Dao. We feel the possibility of the Great Oneness and balance of the tai chi axis.

Practices to Nourish Will, Wisdom and a Balanced Attitude Towards Fear

The forms in this sequence help us draw on our strength of will, wisdom and balanced emotion of fear. The first two are forms found in the Tai Chi Qigong 18 Forms and Eight Silk Brocades respectively. These can be done as part of these sequences, on their own or in this series for working with fear. When I practise and teach these forms, they engender a deep sense of peace and alignment with a source and spirit beyond the physical.

Rowing the Boat in the Centre/Heart of the Lake (*Hu Xin Hua Chuan*)

This form is traditionally the sixth form of the 18 Forms. It works to strengthen the arms, back and kidneys. It also helps open the shoulders and condition the legs. The name is significant: rowing a boat in the centre of a lake brings a quality of gentle, peaceful endurance. If we were rowing along a river rapid, the movements would be hasty and forceful. By placing yourself at the heart of a lake, this means you have already rowed half of your journey. Appreciate the inner reserve, or *zhi*, that has taken you here.

Regular practice of this form helps purify the kidneys, urinary bladder, liver and intestines. It also circulates the blood flow more efficiently in the body, helping us eliminate waste materials and stagnation, and filling it with more vitality and space for the healthy, balanced flow of qi.

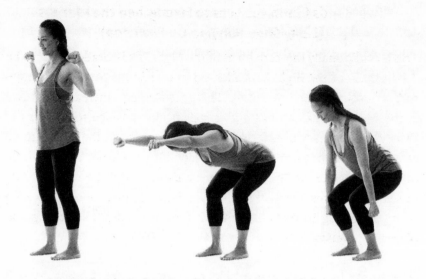

FORM INSTRUCTIONS

1. Start in *Wuji*, taking long, slow, even, fine and deep breaths.

2. Shape the hands as though each is holding an imaginary oar of a boat.

3. Inhale and draw your elbows back, as though you can draw the oars of your boat up out of the water.

4. Exhale and reach both hands forwards, extending the head and spine forward in a straight line. Lower the hips down, and keep the knees bent as you reach the crown of the head away from the tailbone. Then inhale and begin to stand, lowering the hands while they still hold imaginary oars of a boat. This completes one round.

5. Continue, exhaling to reach both hands forward. Repeat this movement of rowing the oars of a boat for 5–9 rounds. As you move your arms, you might imagine how quiet and still you could feel as you gently row the oars of a boat through the waters of a still lake. You can perhaps tap into the quiet endurance and deep peace that are qualities associated with the element of Water. Also sense the calm and clarity that nourishes and feeds your ability to listen and respond with the soft strength of the oars moving through water.

6. When you finish all 5–9 rounds, begin to release the hands and arms down as you stand up.

7. Release the hands from holding the oars into *Wuji*. Observe how you feel.

Two Hands Climb the Legs to Strengthen the Kidneys
(*Liang Shou Pan Jiao Gu Shen Yao*)

This is traditionally the sixth form of the Eight Silk Brocades, and can be done as part of the Eight Brocades, on its own, or as part of this three-part series for Water's emotions. This practice helps increase flexibility in the back and hamstrings and is specifically believed to benefit the kidneys and urinary bladder. It primarily works with the idea that we can draw in essence from the sky and fill it into our body. You can think of essence as the wisdom from your ancestors and the cosmos. The movements in this form are simple, yet, with the intention of working with connecting to our ancestral wisdom, it becomes a moving and powerful practice.

If you have lower back problems, be sure to keep your knees more deeply bent when you fold forward.

FORM INSTRUCTIONS

1. Start in *Wuji*, taking long, slow, even, fine and deep breaths.

2. Place your hands on the lower back, palms open on the kidneys. Take a breath in and, as you breathe out, fold down, tracing the backs of the legs with your hands. This is part of the urinary bladder meridian.

3. Inhale and begin to rise up, tracing the hands smoothly up along the inner legs: this is the kidney meridian line. When you reach the torso, the hands float off the body and lift up towards heaven, the sky. Use your hands to draw down some essence and spirit into the form of your body.

4. Starting with your exhale, begin to draw the hands down, filling with vital essence from the heavens. Earth is believed to give us our blood and bones; heaven, our essence and spirit. Invite the breath to be natural and steady through the descent and filling of essence into your body. Allow the form of the body to be enriched with all these qualities, and specifically feed this essence into your kidneys and bones. This completes one cycle of this form.

5. Inhale and bring your hands once again to the kidneys, palms open, and begin the sequence again. Repeat Steps 2–4 for 5–9 rounds.

6. Do the Closing Form for Peaceful Qi (see page 61): Inhale and gather vital essence from heaven and nourishment for your blood and bones from the

earth in your hands as they reach out to the sides and then overhead. Then turn the palms to face the earth, middle fingers pointing towards each other. Begin to lower the hands down in front of your face, chest and torso, and fill with the qualities of healthy essence and nourishment to feed all aspects of your body, mind and spirit.

7. Finish by placing your hands stacked on the lower *dantian*. Notice how your body feels. Breathe.

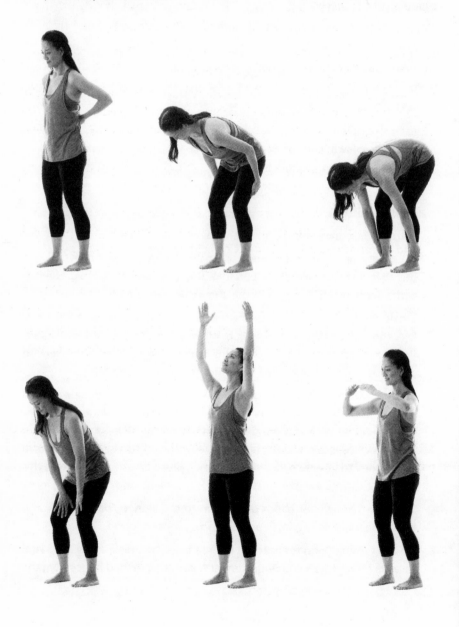

Closing Form for Peaceful Qi
(*An Zhang Ping Qi*)

This simple, classical qigong practice for clearing, gathering and sealing Water uses intention and simple movements to affect the emotions and movement of qi through the body (see page 183).

FORM INSTRUCTIONS

1. Start in *Wuji*, taking long, slow, even, fine and deep breaths.

2. Breathe naturally and with awareness in the *dantian*. Continue this *dantian* breathing throughout the following movements.

3. Turn the palms out and begin to move them slowly and deliberately to the sides and then overhead. As you do this, gather imbalanced *zhi*. This can be excessive wilfulness or, conversely, a lack of will. Also gather qualities of fear out of balance in your body and mind.

4. Once the hands are overhead, turn the palms to face the earth, middle fingers pointing towards each other, elbows bent.

5. Slowly and deliberately begin to lower the hands down in front of your face, neck, chest and belly. Use the intention to clear out imbalanced will and any unhelpful fears you might be holding in your mind and heart.

6. The movement in Steps 3–5 then repeats, with a different intention: gather qualities of Water's emotion and spirit in balance – healthy will and balanced fear. Fill into the space you have cleared.

7. The final movement is to gather all you have filled: healthy will and balanced fear. Seal this into your kidneys and bones to help you nourish your deepest wisdom.

FINAL NOTE

Once you have finished all three movements, remain in *Wuji* for a few breaths and absorb the way you feel. You can complete this by placing your palms on the lower *dantian* and noticing how you feel.

CONCLUSION

Tai Chi Axis and the Dao

The Three Lessons

My journey of qigong began in Beijing over 15 years ago, when I was stressed out and overtired. The fortune I had of meeting qigong and Five Element teachers while living there opened up possibilities for changing my life's trajectory in ways I never would have imagined possible. Now, halfway around the world and nearly half a century old, I cannot imagine what my life or health would be like without these practices.

In the years that I have studied and taught qigong, I have learned three main things. The first is that **qigong supports us best when we lean away from extremes**. As the *Dao De Jing* writes,

> Fill your bowl to the brim
> and it will spill.
> Keep sharpening your knife
> and it will blunt.
> Chase after money and security
> and your heart will never unclench.
> Care about people's approval
> and you will be their prisoner.
>
> Do your work, then step back.
> The only path to serenity.

Dao de Jing (Tao Te Ching), Chapter 9[1]

Qigong is a middle-path practice. We use movement and breath to nourish our health and bring balance to the body so that our mind, heart and spirit can experience an enriching and peaceful life. This means that we do not push the body towards extremes or neglect it and let it decay. It also means that we work with intentions that support rather than deplete our resources. We fill our bowl so that we can enjoy a drink without the risk of it spilling over. We sharpen our knife so that it cuts well but does not blunt. We pursue goals that allow our hearts to remain spacious and open rather than crowded, tight and clenched. We simply do that which allows us to live with greater clarity, kindness and compassion towards ourselves and others. We do our work, step back, and take a step on the path towards serenity.

The second thing I have learned is that **qigong has enabled me to feel a deep respect for nature and therefore of my own body**. It has allowed me to cultivate greater awareness of myself and my relationship with the natural world. This perspective has helped me and my students remember that all that is around us is also always within us. Knowing that my elemental make-up is mirrored in the natural world makes me feel that I can stand firmly with my feet on the earth and my head towards the heavens. It opens me up to the feeling of the tai chi axis, present and aligned.

The tai chi axis is how each of us may physically begin to experience the wholeness and Oneness of tai chi – understood to be the Supreme Ultimate or Great Pole. Understanding the essence of tai chi is difficult. Most simply put, tai chi is the potential and space of *wuji* that gives rise to the harmonious movement of yin and yang; in turn generating the Five Elements. Yet the Five Elements also create yin and yang, which give rise to *Wuji*. In essence, everything is one and the same. It is part of the Dao, which the *Dao De Jing* describes as what 'cannot be seen' and 'cannot be heard' yet 'cannot be exhausted by use'.[2]

The Dao is the Way. It is 'great', and considered to be the 'mother of all worlds',[3] but also humble and low like a clod of earth.[4] Though impossible to grasp, it can be directly experienced through meditative practices such as those qigong offers. In one of the most ancient Daoist texts, dating back to approximately 300 BCE, we are told: 'Cultivate your mind, make your thoughts tranquil, and the Way can thereby be attained.'[5] By investing into practices that optimised their health, balance and harmony, the ancient Daoists believed they could experience the Dao.

This brings me to the third and perhaps most important thing I have learned: **we are all part of something more than just ourselves which is fluid and always changing**. I believe that this is the Dao. The famous Han Dynasty historian Sima Qian described how the Dao 'shifts with the times and changes in response to things…The general drift of its teaching is simple and easy to hold onto: much is achieved with little effort.'[6]

As qigong's roots are in Daoism, this idea that it can shift with the times and change in response to things has helped me maintain a balance between staying true to tradition, while also being open to new methods and approaches to learning. I value learning set qigong forms and believe practising them accurately is important. I also equally recognise that the moment anyone – myself included – becomes too rigid or dictatorial about how forms should be done, then the ability to shift and respond is potentially lost. This resistance may undermine the very essence of the Dao, which is *wuwei* – the effortless effort that allows us to flow the way the river flows.

That said, following forms and adhering to methodology and structure should come first. We must practise and learn technique. But paraphrasing something Bruce Lee once said, we should aim to learn technique, practise technique, then forget technique. For myself, this means that once I have an understanding of certain concepts, there is the freedom to break from them. For myself, I am still learning techniques every day. My hope, however, is that one day I might do as John Coltrane does with his saxophone: bust through form to play off the horn. His music transcends traditional structure but nevertheless produces sounds many consider masterful. For myself, the freedom within qigong to be innovative is imperative. It is how the 7000 forms alive today may continue to grow and be created out of the formlessness and Oneness of the Dao.

I hope that by reading this book you have been inspired to continue to learn about qigong and develop practices that can be authentically integrated into your life. I also hope that the principles that underlie qigong grant you the same possibilities for better health, balance and peace that the practice has brought to mine and my students' lives.

Lastly, as you continue to practise qigong, it can be helpful to remember these wise words from the *Dao De Jing*: 'The giant pine tree grows from a tiny sprout' and 'The journey of a thousand miles starts from beneath your feet'. We always begin from where we are, and only then can we travel far with a full and nourished life. To make this journey of a thousand miles, qigong grants us a map and compass that can help us navigate life's unpredictable roads and steer us gently towards a place of contentment and peace.

Any journey, regardless of distance, always starts from beneath your feet.

ADDITIONAL PRACTICE GUIDE

In addition to practising qigong in the short element-focused sequences I have outlined in this book, you may also choose to practise complete sequences for the Five Elements, Five Animal Frolics (*Wu Qin Xi*), Eight Silk Brocades (*Baduanjin*), Tai Chi Qigong 18 Forms (*Shibashi*) and the Five Element Mudra practices. If you would like to practise these as complete sequences, the orders are provided here.

For the Five Element Forms, Five Element Mudras, Eight Silk Brocades (*Baduanjin*) and Tai Chi Qigong 18 Forms (*Shibashi*), you can also refer to my DVD and digital download of Qigong Basics and Qigong Flow, available on Vimeo and Amazon.

Five Element Forms

These forms can be done starting with Wood or Metal: Wood for energy and creation; Metal for connecting more to inspiration, breath and spirit.

OPTION SEQUENCE ONE

- **Wood**: for the liver and gall bladder   *pages 48–50*
- **Fire**: for the heart   *pages 75–7*
- **Earth**: for the stomach and spleen   *pages 121–2*
- **Metal**: for the lungs and large intestine   *pages 170–2*
- **Water**: for the kidneys and urinary bladder   *pages 212–4*

OPTION SEQUENCE TWO

- **Metal**: for the lungs and large intestine   *pages 170–2*
- **Water**: for the kidneys and urinary bladder   *pages 212–4*
- **Wood**: for the liver and gall bladder   *pages 48–50*
- **Fire**: for the heart   *pages 75–7*
- **Earth**: for the stomach and spleen   *pages 121–2*

Five Element Mudras

Like the Five Element Forms above, these mudras can also be done starting with Wood or Metal.

OPTION SEQUENCE ONE

- **Wood**: for the liver and gall bladder   *pages 60–1*
- **Fire**: for the heart   *pages 95–7 and 103–4*
- **Earth**: for the stomach and spleen   *pages 141–2*
- **Metal**: for the lungs and large intestine   *pages 179–82*
- **Water**: for the kidneys and urinary bladder   *pages 196–7*

OPTION SEQUENCE TWO

- **Metal**: for the lungs and large intestine   *pages 179–82*
- **Water**: for the kidneys and urinary bladder   *pages 196–7*
- **Wood**: for the liver and gall bladder   *pages 60–1*
- **Fire**: for the heart   *pages 95–7 and 103–4*
- **Earth**: for the stomach and spleen   *pages 141–2*

Five Animal Frolics

If practising these forms in a sequence, the traditional method and order are different from those of the Five Element Forms and Mudras. It is believed that the Crane, when practised first, creates a warm-up for the whole system by opening the spine and the major meridians that connect through the body. The second form, Bear, develops energy and strength in our body and connects us to our essence, or *jing*. The Monkey is next as it builds quickness and agility. The Deer stretches the spine and legs. The Tiger is last as it is the most formidable of the animals, and is the most dynamic of the practices.

1. **Crane** (nourishes Fire and the heart) *pages 83–5*
2. **Bear** (nourishes Water and the kidneys) *pages 208–10*
3. **Monkey** (nourishes Earth and the spleen) *pages 116–8*
4. **Deer** (nourishes Wood and the liver) *pages 52–6*
5. **Tiger** (nourishes Metal and the lungs) *pages 158–61*

Eight Silk Brocades (*Baduanjin*)

This order of the Eight Brocades varies slightly from the traditional ordering, in that I have chosen to switch the second and third forms. In most Eight Brocade practices, Opening the Bow to Let the Arrow Fly comes second, and Raise the Hands to Condition the Stomach and Spleen third. However, I find that when I perform Raise the Hands to Condition the Stomach and Spleen before Opening the Bow to Let the Arrow Fly, I feel more integrated in my centre and able to use my bow with better intention and aim.

1. **Two Hands Support the Heavens for the Triple Heater**
   (*Shuang Shou Qing Tian Li San Jiao*) *pages 94–5*

2. **Raise the Hands to Condition the Stomach and Spleen**
   (*Tiao Li Pi Wei Dan Ju Shou*) *pages 133–4*

3. **Opening the Bow to Let the Arrow Fly**
   (*Zuo You Kai Gong Si She Diao*) *pages* 50–1

4. **Looking Backwards to Eliminate Five Fatigues and Seven Illnesses**
   (*Wu Lao Qi Shang Xiang Hou Qiao*) *pages* 123–4

5. **Nod the Head and Wag the Tail to Calm Heart Fire**
   (*Yao Tou Bai Wei Qu Xin Huo*) *pages* 81–2

6. **Two Hands Climb the Legs to Strengthen the Kidneys**
   (*Liang Shou Pan Jiao Gu Shen Yao*) *pages* 221–2

7. **Punching with an Angry Gaze to Increase Strength**
   (*Wo Quan Nu Mu Zeng Li Qi*) *pages* 58–9

8. **Shake the Back Seven Times to Eliminate the 100 Illnesses**
   (*Bei Hou Qi Dian Bai Bing Xiao*) *pages* 174–5

Tai Chi Qigong 18 Forms (*Taiji Qigong Shibashi*)

This sequence has a set order, but as I have practised this over the years, I have changed the order very slightly from the original so that it feels more fluid in my body. The following order is the one I tend to practise and teach.

1. **Pulsing/Harmonising the Qi** (*Qi Shi Tiao Xi*) *pages* 41–2

2. **Opening the Chest** (*Kai Kuo Xiong Huai*) *pages* 74–5

3. **Separating Clouds** (*Lun Bi Fen Yun*) *pages* 86–7

4. **Rainbow Dance** (*Hui Wu Cai Hong*) *pages* 134–6

5. **Rolling Ball** (*Ding Bu Dao Juan Gong*) *pages* 42–3

6. **Rowing the Boat in the Centre of the Lake** (*Hu Xin Hua Chuan*)
   pages 219–20

7. **Lifting Ball** (*Jian Qian Tuo Qiu*) *pages* 101–2

NOTES

INTRODUCTION

1 Keown, D., *The Spark in the Machine*, 2014: pp. 31, 78.
2 Cohen, K., *The Way of Qigong*, 1997: p. 18.
3 Gallagher, P., *History of the Later Han Dynasty*, in *Drawing Silk: Masters' Secrets for Successful Tai Chi Practice*, 2008: p. 2.
4 Translation by Stephen Mitchell, *Tao Te Ching: A New English Version*, 2006: Chapter 64.

PART I
WOOD ELEMENT: NOURISHING OUR ROOTS

1 Dechar, L., *Five Spirits: Alchemical Acupuncture for Psychological and Spiritual Healing*, 2006: p. 195.
2 The forms are based on the tai chi Yang-style Forms. First developed in Shanghai in 1982 by tai chi chuan masters He Weiqi and Lin Housheng, these forms are a fusion of tai chi's fluid, even movements with qigong's meditative and breath-focused qualities. The 18 Forms are now practised by millions of people around the world.
3 Ishida, H., 'Body and Mind: The Chinese Perspective', in *Taoist Meditation and Longevity Techniques*, edited by Livia Kohn, 1989: pp. 49–50.
4 Diabetes Self Management, 2014: 'Nighttime Hypoglycemia'. Available online at https://www.diabetesselfmanagement.com/diabetes-resources/definitions/nighttime-hypoglycemia/
5 Cohen, K., op cit, pp. 199–211.
6 Ishida, H., op cit, p. 50.
7 Confucius: *The Analects*, XII.22.

PART 2
FIRE ELEMENT: NOURISHING THE HEART

1 Kohn, L., 'Guarding the One', in *Taoist Meditation and Longevity Techniques,* op cit, p. 127.

2 Keown, D., op cit, p. 128.

3 Zhang Jiebin (1563–c.1650), a Ming Dynasty commentator who was influential in Chinese medicine. Translated by Claude Larre and Elisabeth Rochat de la Vallée, *Rooted in Spirit: The Heart of Chinese Medicine,* 1995: p. 46.

4 'Heart attacks "worse in the morning"', 28 April 2011. NHS.com. Available at https://www.nhs.uk/news/heart-and-lungs/heart-attacks-worse-in-the-morning/ [Accessed 23 April 2018].

5 Cohen, K., op cit, p. 235.

6 Ibid, p. 200.

7 Dechar, L., op cit, p. 42.

8 Larre, C. and Rochat de la Vallée, E., op cit, p. 170.

9 Ibid.

PART 3
EARTH ELEMENT: NOURISHING THE MIND

1 *The Natural World.* Han Dynasty text (206BCE–220CE). Translated by Eva Wong, *Being Doaist: Wisdom for Living a Balanced Life,* 2015: p. 40

2 Cohen, K., op cit, p. 161.

3 *Monkey: The Journey to the West.* Translated from the Chinese by Arthur Waley, 2005: p. 26. [Kindle for Mac.] Retrieved from Amazon.co.uk.

4 Porter, B., *Road to Heaven: Encounters with Chinese Hermits,* 1993: p. 18.

5 Hucker, C., *China's Imperial Past: An Introduction to Chinese History and Culture,* 1975: p. 143.

6 Some contemporary practitioners of Chinese medicine refer to the spleen as the Spleen-Pancreas, as the function of the spleen in Chinese medicine overlaps with the function of the pancreas. See Keown, D., op cit, p. 183.

7 Staughton, J., 'Can You Live Without a Stomach?', 2017. Scienceabc.com [online]. Available at https://www.scienceabc.com/humans/can-you-live-without-a-stomach.html [Accessed 8 May 2018].

8 Despeux, C., 'Gymnastics: The Ancient Tradition', in *Taoist Meditation and Longevity Techniques,* op cit, p. 226.

PART 4

METAL ELEMENT: NOURISHING THE SPIRIT

1 Ralph Waldo Emerson (1803–1882), *The Complete Works, Vol. X: Lectures and Biographical Sketches*, 1904. Available online at Bartley.com https://www.bartleby.com/90/1005.html.

2 Online Etymology Dictionaries. Available at https://www.etymonline.com/word/inspiration [Accessed 14 May 2018].

3 *Phaedo*, 66C-D, translated by David Gallop, in John M. Dillon, 'Rejecting the Body, Refining the Body: Some Remarks on the Development of Plantonist Asceticism', 1998, in *Asceticism*, edited by Vincent L. Wimbush and Richard Valantasis.

4 *Maitreya Upaniṣad*, in Patrick Olivelle, 'Deconstruction of the Body in Indian Asceticism', 1998, in *Asceticism*, edited by Vincent L. Wimbush and Richard Valantasis, pp. 188–210.

5 Ibid.

6 Murck, A., *Poetry and Painting in Song China: The Subtle Art of Dissent*, 2000: p. 75. Wilder, G.D. and Ingram, J.H., *Analysis of Chinese Characters* (Second Edition), 1972: p. 361.

7 Reichstein, G., *Wood Becomes Water*, 1998: p. 136.

8 Ibid.

9 *Neijing Suwen*, Chapter 8 of the *Yellow Emperor's Classic of Internal Medicine*. Translated by Larre, C., and Rochat de la Vallée, E., in *The Secret Treatise of the Spiritual Orchid*, 2003: p. 49.

10 Keown, D., op cit, p. 172.

11 Lewis, D., *The Tao of Natural Breathing: For Health, Well-Being and Inner Growth*, 2006: p.42 [Kindle for Mac.] Retrieved from Amazon.co.uk.

12 Keown, D. op cit, p. 170.

PART 5

WATER ELEMENT: NOURISHING OUR DEEPEST WISDOM

1 Ghorsh, P., 'Why do we sleep?', 15 May 2015. BBC news online. Available at http://www.bbc.co.uk/news/science-environment-32606341 [Accessed 28 May 2018].

2 Primarily, water acts as a solvent: it breaks down waste and then transports nutrients to where they are needed for growth.

3 Book of Genesis 1:1–6.

4 *Ṛgveda* 1.32.4, in Brown, N., 'The Creation Myth of the Ṛgveda', in *Journal of the American Oriental Society*, Vol. 62, No. 2, (June 1942): pp. 85–98. [pdf] Published by: American Oriental Society. Available at http://www.jstor.org/stable/594460 [Accessed: 12 August 2016].

5 Book of Genesis 6–9.

6 *Tao Te Ching: A New English Version*, op cit, Chapter 78.

7 The simplified version of this character is 听, which does not show the richness of the original context.

8 Tillich, P., *Love, Power, and Justice: Ontological Analyses and Ethical Applications*, 1954: p. 84.

9 Davis, R., *Qigong Through the Seasons*, 2015: pp. 216–217.

10 *Taoist Meditation and Longevity Techniques*, op cit.

11 Larre, C., and Rochat de la Vallée, E., *Rooted in Spirit*, op cit, p. 147.

12 Keown, D., op cit, pp. 142–3 and Reichstein. G., op cit, pp. 180–81.

13 'Why the "Stress Hormone" is Public Enemy No. 1: 5 simple ways to lower your cortisol levels without drugs', 2013. *Psychology Today* online. Available at https://www.psychologytoday.com/us/blog/the-athletes-way/201301/cortisol-why-the-stress-hormone-is-public-enemy-no-1 [Accessed 29 May 2018].

14 Jarret, L.S., *The Clinical Practice of Chinese Medicine*, 2003: p. 376.

CONCLUSION:
TAI CHI AXIS AND THE DAO

1 *Tao Te Ching: A New English Version*, op cit. 2006.

2 *Lao Tzu Tao Te Ching*, XXXV, 1963: p. 40. Translated by D.C. Lau.

3 Ibid, XXV: 56–56a, p. 82.

4 Creel, H.G., 'The Great Clod', in *What is Taoism? And Other Studies in Chinese Cultural History*, 1970: p. 34.

5 *Nei-yeh (Inward Training)* V:13–14, in *Original Tao: Inward Training and the Foundations of Taoist Mysticism*, p. 54. Translated by Harold D. Roth.

6 *The History of the Han*, in 'The Frustration of the Second Confucius' [pdf] Available at http://www.sunypress.edu/pdf/53296.pdf [Accessed 29 May 2018].

BIBLIOGRAPHY

Brown, N., 1942. 'The Creation Myth of the Rig Veda', in *Journal of the American Oriental Society*, Vol. 62, No. 2 (June, 1942). [pdf] Published by: American Oriental Society. Available at http://www.jstor.org/stable/594460.

Cohen, K., 1997. *The Way of Qigong: The Art and Science of Chinese Energy Healing*. New York: Ballantine Books.

Confucius: The Analects (Lun yü). Translated with an introduction by D.C. Lau, 1979. London: Penguin Books.

Creel, H.G., 1970. 'The Great Clod'. In H.G. Creel. *What is Taoism? And Other Studies in Chinese Cultural History*. Chicago – London: University of Chicago Press.

Davis, R., 2015. *Qigong Through the Seasons: How to Stay Healthy All Year Long with Qigong, Meditation, Diet and Herbs*. London and Philadelphia: Singing Dragon.

Dechar, L.E., 2006. *Five Spirits: Alchemical Acupuncture for Psychological and Spiritual Healing*. New York: Lantern Books.

Despeux, C., 1989. 'Gymnastics: The Ancient Tradition', in *Taoist Meditation and Longevity Techniques*, edited by Livia Kohn. Ann Arbour: Center for Chinese Studies, The University of Michigan.

Gallagher, P.B., 2008. *Drawing Silk: Masters' Secrets for Successful Tai Chi Practice*. Fairview, North Carolina: Total Tai Chi

Huandi Neijing Lingshu (The Yellow Emperor's Classic of Internal Medicine). Translated from Chinese by Claude Larre, S.J. and Elisabeth Rochat de la Vallée; translated from French by Sarah Stang. Barrytown, New York: Station Hill Press.

Huang Ti Nei Cing Su Wen: The Yellow Emperor's Classic of Internal Medicine. Chapters 1–34. Translated from the Chinese with an Introductory Study by Ilza Veith. 1975. Oakland, California: University of California Press.

Hucker, C., 1975. *China's Imperial Past: An Introduction to Chinese History and Culture*. Stanford, California: Stanford University Press.

Ishida, H., 1987. 'Body and Mind: The Chinese Perspective'. In L. Kohn, ed. 1989. *Taoist Meditation and Longevity Techniques*. Ann Arbor, MI: Center for Chinese Studies, The University of Michigan.

Jarret, L.S., 2003. *The Clinical Practice of Chinese Medicine*. Stockbridge, Massachusetts: Spirit Path Press.

Keown, D., 2014. *The Spark in the Machine: How the Science of Acupuncture Explains the Mysteries of Western Medicine*. London: Singing Dragon.

Kohn, L., 1989. 'Guarding the One', in *Taoist Meditation and Longevity Techniques*, edited by Livia Kohn. Ann Arbor: Center for Chinese Studies, The University of Michigan.

Kohn, L., 2008. *Chinese Healing Exercises: The Tradition of Daoyin*. Honolulu: University of Hawai'i Press.

Lao Tzu Tao Te Ching, 1963. Translated by D.C. Lau. London: Penguin Books Ltd.

Larre, C. and Vallée, E. R., 1992. *Rooted in Spirit: The Heart of Chinese Medicine – A sinological interpretation of Chapter Eight of Huandi Neijing Lingshu*. Translated from French by Sarah Stang. Barrytown, New York: Station Hill Press.

Larre, C. and Vallée, E. R., 2003. *The Secret Treatise of the Spiritual Orchid: Neijing Suwen Chapter 8*. London: Monkey Press.

Lewis, D., 2006. *The Tao of Natural Breathing: For Health, Well-Being and Inner Growth*. [Kindle for Mac.] Boulder: Shambala.

Maitreya Upaniṣad, in Patrick Olivelle, 'Deconstruction of the Body in Indian Asceticism', 1998, in *Asceticism*, edited by Vincent L. Wimbush and Richard Valantasis. New York: Oxford University Press.

Monkey: The Journey to the West. Translated from the Chinese by Arthur Waley, 2005. [Kindle for Mac.]

Murck, A., 2000. *Poetry and Painting in Song China: The Subtle Art of Dissent*. Cambridge and London: Harvard University Asia Center for the Harvard-Yenching Institute.

Nei-yeh (Inward Training) V:13–14, translated by Harold D. Roth, 1999, in *Original Tao: Inward Training and the Foundations of Taoist Mysticism*. New York; Chichester: Columbia University Press.

Phaedo, 66C-D, translated by David Gallop, in John M. Dillon, 1998, 'Rejecting the Body, Refining the Body: Some Remarks on the Development of Plantonist Asceticism' in *Asceticism*, edited by Vincent L. Wimbush and Richard Valantasis. Oxford: Oxford University Press.

Porter, B., 1993. *Road to Heaven: Encounters with Chinese Hermits*. San Francisco: Mercury House.

Reichstein, G., 1998. *Wood Becomes Water: Chinese Medicine in Everyday Life.* New York: Kodansha America, Inc.

Tao Te Ching: A New English Version. Translation by Stephen Mitchell, 2006. New York: Harper Perennial Modern Classics.

Taoist Meditation and Longevity Techniques, 1989. Edited by Livia Kohn. Ann Arbor: Center for Chinese Studies, The University of Michigan.

Wilder, G.D. and Ingram, J.H., 1972. *Analysis of Chinese Characters* (Second Edition). New York: Dove Publications.

Wong, E., 2015. *Being Taoist: Wisdom for Living a Balanced Life.* Boston and London: Shambala Publications, Ltd.

Wu Qin Xi: Five-Animal Qigong Exercises. 2008. Compiled by the Chinese Health Qigong Association. London and Philadelphia: Singing Dragon.

The Yellow Emperor's Classic of Medicine: A New Translation of the Neijing Suwen with Commentary. Naoshing Ni, PhD. 1995. Boulder: Shambala.

Yin, H.H. and Shuai, H.C., 1992. *Fundamentals of Traditional Chinese Medicine.* Beijing, China: Foreign Languages Press.

ACKNOWLEDGEMENTS

I would first like to thank my parents for their commitment to keeping Chinese culture and ideas alive as I grew up in the milieu of the American landscape. Throughout their lives they aspired to become bridges between China and the West, and always encouraged myself and my brothers to be the same.

I am also deeply grateful to my mentors, teachers and academic professors: Erich Schiffmann, Donna Farhi, Sifu Matthew Cohen, Cameron Tukapua, Martin Aylward, Max Strom, Dr Antonello Palumbo, Dr Ulrich Pagel and Dr Ted Profers. They have encouraged me to explore my passion for qigong, philosophy and the healing arts with a balance of enthusiasm, humility, commitment and a healthy grain of salt. Many thanks as well to my editor, Olivia Morris, and my literary agent, Anna Hogarty; their enthusiasm in bringing qigong to wider audiences made writing this book possible.

Lastly, I would like to thank triyoga and my students for supporting my work; James Rafael, who reviewed early versions of this book; Sylvie Minois for her stunning illustrations; and Aaron Deemer for all the photos that accompany my text. As my better half, Aaron also deserves a special, final acknowledgement. His humour, love, support and kindness inspire me to better live the teachings that I hope to share.

ABOUT THE AUTHOR

Mimi Kuo-Deemer is dedicated to sharing the ways in which qigong and other healing arts can help people meet the messy, complicated job of being human with greater awareness, compassion and ease. She is a teacher of both students and of other teachers, having practised and taught for over 20 years in China, the UK, Europe and the United States. In 1994, she graduated from Stanford University and in 2016, she received an MA with distinction from SOAS in Traditions of Yoga and Meditation. Originally from Tucson, Arizona, she lived in China for over 14 years where she worked as a photojournalist as well acted as co-founder and co-director of Yoga Yard, Beijing's first and leading yoga studio. Mimi now lives in the UK, where she is a senior teacher at triyoga, London's pre-eminent centre for health and wellbeing. *Qigong and the Tai Chi Axis: Nourishing Practices for Body, Mind and Spirit* is her first book.

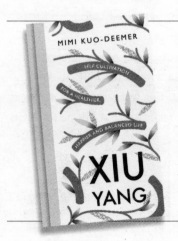

ALSO BY MIMI

In this nurturing lifestyle guide, Mimi Kuo-Deemer champions the contemporary value of adopting this ancient approach. Through a combination of practices from meditation and mindfulness to yoga and qigong, *Xiu Yang* offers a fresh approach to finding balance and bringing peace into your life, home and community.